OPCS Surveys of Psychiatric
Morbidity in Great Britain

Report 2

Physical complaints, service use and treatment of adults with psychiatric disorders

Howard Meltzer
Baljit Gill
Mark Petticrew
Kerstin Hinds

London: HMSO

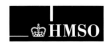

Published by HMSO and available from:

HMSO Publications Centre
(Mail, fax and telephone orders only)
PO Box 276, London SW8 5DT
Telephone orders 0171 873 9090
General enquiries 0171 873 0011
(queuing system in operation for both numbers)
Fax orders 0171 873 8200

HMSO Bookshops
49 High Holborn, London WC1V 6HB
(counter service only)
0171 873 0011 Fax 0171 831 1326
68–69 Bull Street, Birmingham B4 6AD
0121 236 9696   Fax 0121 236 9699
33 Wine Street, Bristol BS1 2BQ
0117 9264306 Fax 0117 9294515
9–21 Princess Street, Manchester M60 8AS
0161 834 7201 Fax 0161 833 0634
16 Arthur Street, Belfast BT1 4GD
01232 238451 Fax 01232 235401
71 Lothian Road, Edinburgh EH3 9AZ
0131 228 4181 Fax 0131 229 2734
The HMSO Oriel Bookshop
The Friary, Cardiff CF1 4AA
01222 395548 Fax 01222 384347

HMSO's Accredited Agents
(see Yellow Pages)

and through good booksellers

List of tables

Page

Chapter 1: Characteristics of adults with neurotic disorders

1.1 Proportion of all adults with each disorder, and the primary disorder distribution by sex   7

1.2 Percentage of people with each disorder by sex   7

1.3 Number of neurotic disorders by disorder and sex   8

1.4 Comorbidity among neurotic disorders by sex   9

1.5 CIS-R scores of those with different neurotic disorders   10

1.6 CIS-R scores by the number of neurotic disorders   10

1.7 Age, ethnicity, marital status and family unit type by neurotic disorder and sex   11

1.8 Educational qualifications, Social class, employment status and tenure by neurotic disorder and sex   14

1.9 Region, country and locality by neurotic disorder and sex   17

1.10 The prevalence of symptons measured on the CIS-R by neurotic disorder   20

1.11 How long people had been experiencing the symptoms involved in the diagnosis of neurotic disorders   20

1.12 Severity of limiting effects of symptoms by neurotic disorder   21

Chapter 2: Neurotic disorders and physical complaints

2.1 Percentage of adults with each physical complaint by neurotic disorder, compared with the 1989 GHS estimates   29

2.2 Long-standing physical complaints by age (grouped) by whether had a neurotic disorder and sex   30

2.3 Long-standing physical complaints by number of neurotic disorders and sex   33

2.4 Long-standing physical complaints by neurotic disorder and sex   34

2.5 Odds ratios of each long-standing physical complaint associated with having a neurotic disorder   35

2.6 Number of neurotic disorders by long-standing physical complaint and sex   36

2.7 Cumulative CIS-R scores for worry about physical health by long-standing physical complaint   37

Chapter 3: Medication and other forms of treatment

3.1 Type of treatment by number of neurotic disorders   41

3.2 Type of treatment by type of neurotic disorder   41

3.3 Type of medication by number of neurotic disorders   42

3.4 Type of therapy or counselling by number of neurotic disorders   42

3.5 Odds ratios associated with treatment by antidepressants   42

3.6 Odds ratios associated with treatment by anxiolytics of hypnotics   42

3.7 Odds ratios associated with treatment by any medication   43

3.8 Odds ratios associated with treatment by counselling   43

3.9 Odds ratios associated with treatment by therapy   43

3.10 Odds ratios associated with treatment by counselling or therapy   43

3.11 Type of medication taken by adults with neurotic disorders who also have physical illness   44

Chapter 4: Use of services

4.1 GP consultations by presence of neurotic disorder and sex 52

4.2 Reasons for consultations on own behalf by individuals with neurotic disorders during past two weeks 53

4.3 Odds ratios of socio-demographic correlates of GP consultations for any reason in past two weeks 53

4.4 Odds ratios of socio-demographic correlates of GP consultations for physical complaint in past year 54

4.5 Odds ratios of socio-demographic correlates of GP consultations for a mental problem in past year 54

4.6 Percentage of people with neurotic disorders who had been in-patients in past year, and reason for in-patient stay 55

4.7 Number of separate in-patient stays in past 12 months among people with neurotic disorders 55

4.8 Person seen by patient when in hospital for mental health problem 55

4.9 Number of places visited as out-patient or day patient in past year 55

4.10 Reasons for out-patient or day patient visits by people with neurotic disorders during the past year 56

4.11 Type of place visited by out-patients and day patients for a mental health problen in past year 56

4.12 Person normally seen at hospital/clinic by people eith neurotic disorders when visiting because of mental health problems 56

4.13 Source of help which had been turned down by people with neurotic disorders 57

4.14 Reason for turning down help or support 57

4.15 Reason for not seeing a doctor or other professional when others thought they should 57

Chapter 5: Adults with a psychotic disorder

5.1 Socio-demographic characteristics of adults with a psychotic disorder 59

5.2 Characteristics of adults with a psychotic disorder compared 1with those with a neurotic disorder and those without a mental disorder 60

5.3 Prevalence of CIS-R symptoms by type of mental disorder 60

5.4 Medication and treatment received by those with a psychotic disorder 61

5.5 Service use profile 61

Chapter 6: Adults with suicidal thoughts

6.1 Socio-demographic characteristics of adults with suicidal thoughts 63

6.2 Characteristics of adults with suicidal thoughts compared with those with a neurotic disorder and without a mental disorder 64

6.3 Depressive ideas of those with suicidal thoughts 64

6.4 Prevalence of CIS-R symptoms of those with suicidal thoughts 65

6.5 Proportion of adults with suicidal thoughts having each neurotic disorder 65

6.6 Medication and treatment received by those with suicidal thoughts 66

6.7 Service use profile 66

List of figures

Page

Chapter 1:   Characteristics of adults with neurotic disorders
1.1   Proportion of adults with each neurotic disorder(base = adults with any neurotic
     disorder)   2
1.2   CIS-R scores of adults with each neurotic disorder   3

Chapter 2:   Neurotic disorders and physical complaints
2.1   Percentage of adults with each long-standing physical complaint by neurotic disorder   23
2.2   Percentage of adults having any long-standing physical complaint by whether
     had a neurotic disorder and age (grouped)   24
2.3   Percentage of adults having any long-standing physical complaint by the number
     of neurotic disorders and sex   25
2.4   Odds ratios of having each long-standing physical complaint associated with a neurotic
     disorder   26
2.5   The number of neurotic disorders among adults with each type of long-standing
     physical complaint, by sex   27

Chapter 4:   Use of services
4.1   GP consultations on own behalf in past two weeks by people with neurotic disorders,
     by type of disorder   46
4.2   In-patient stays during the past year among people with neurotic disorders, by
     sex and type of disorder   48
4.3   Profile of service use in past year among people with neurotic disorders   51

Notes

Tables showing percentages

The row or column percentages may add to 99% or 101% because of rounding.

The varying positions of the percentage signs and bases in the tables denote the presentation of different types of information. Where there is a percentage sign at the head of a column and the base at the foot, the whole distribution is presented and the individual percentages add to between 99% and 101%. Where there is no percentage sign in the table and a note above the figures, the figures refer to the proportion of people who had the attribute being discussed, and the complementary proportion, to add to 100%, is not shown in the table.

Standard errors are shown in brackets beside percentages in the tables.

The following conventions have been used within tables showing percentages:

-	no cases
0	values less than 0.5%
[ ]	the numbers inside the square brackets are the actual number of observations when the total number of cases, that is the base, is fewer than 30.

Small bases

Very small bases have been avoided wherever possible because of the relatively high sampling errors that attach to small numbers. Often where the numbers are not large enough to justify the use of all categories, classifications have been condensed. However, an item within a classification is occasionally shown separately, even though the base is small, because to combine it with another large category would detract from the value of the larger category. In general, percentage distributions are shown if the base is 30 or more. Where the base is slightly lower, actual numbers are shown in square brackets

Significant differences

The bases for some subgroups presented in the tables were small such that the standard errors around estimates for these groups are biased. Confidence intervals which take account of these biased standard errors were calculated and, although they are not presented in the tables, they were used in testing for statistically significant differences. Statistical significance is explained in Appendix B to this Report.

Focus of the report and survey definitions

Focus of the report

This report is the second of three to look at data from the private household survey of the OPCS surveys of psychiatric morbidity in Great Britain.[1] The report focuses mainly on those with neurotic disorders. Those with a psychotic disorder have been excluded from consideration in all but one chapter owing to the very different nature of their mental illness: Chapter 5 is dedicated to this group.

This report considers:

- the socio-demographic characteristics of those with different disorders

- the relationship between CIS-R scores[2] and neurotic disorders and the comorbidity of neurotic disorders

- the relationships between physical health problems and neurotic and psychotic illnesses

- the medication and other forms of treatment received by those with psychiatric disorders

- the use of services, including consultations with GPs, in-patient stays and out-patient attendances and domiciliary visits

A separate chapter is also included on individuals who were identified as having suicidal thoughts (Chapter 6).

Other reports on the private household survey

Report 1

Report 1, published in May 1995, detailed the prevalence of neurotic symptoms and neurotic and psychotic disorders in the general population. It showed that prevalence of symptoms and disorders varied according to a number of personal, social, and economic characteristics, such as sex, marital status, working status and social class. Report 1 also reported on the prevalence of alcohol and drug dependence.

As the first report on the private household survey, Report 1 also included information on the survey methodology: the sample design, response and the method used to weight the data. The questionnaires used in the survey were printed as an Appendix to Report 1.

Report 3

This report compares adults with and without neurotic and psychotic disorders over a range of measures. These include difficulties associated with mental disorders in respect of activities of daily living, employment, social functioning and finances. Information is also presented on recent stressful life events and the use of tobacco, alcohol and drugs.

Survey definitions

The measures of psychiatric morbidity used in this Report

Ten neurotic disorders are identified in this report. They are:

- mixed anxiety and depressive disorder
- Generalised Anxiety Disorder
- mild, moderate and severe depressive episode (collectively grouped as depressive episode for many analyses)
- agoraphobia, social phobia and specific isolated phobia (individuals could only have one of these and they are combined as 'phobia' for much analysis)

– Obsessive-Compulsive Disorder

– panic disorder

The way in which each of these disorders was identified is shown in Appendix A. It is worth noting here that mixed anxiety and depressive disorder was a catch-all category for adults with a neurotic disorder who were not diagnosed as having one of the other nine disorders identified. This means that while people could have more than one of the other disorders, mixed anxiety and depression was only ever present on its own.

The chapter on psychotic disorders groups together all adults found to have any psychotic illness as the prevalence of these disorders was very low. The way in which psychotic disorders were identified is shown in Appendix A.

When looking at neurotic disorders in this Report, every individual with each disorder is included. This differs from the use of the primary disorder hierarchy used in Report 1 to produce prevalence estimates.[3] Nevertheless, Chapter 1 does include a comparison of the percentage of people with each disorder as their primary disorder and the percentage of people with each disorder. Those with a psychotic

disorder are excluded from the chapters covering neurotic disorders.

This report presents no information about the 316 interviews conducted by proxy as neurotic diagnoses could not be obtained for this group.

Notes and references

1   The private household survey involved interviews with 10,000 randomly sampled adults in Great Britain. In addition to the private household survey, interviews were also conducted in institutions specifically catering for people with mental illness as well as among the homeless.

2   Lewis, G. and Pelosi, A.J., *Manual of the Revised Clinical Interview Schedule, (CIS-R)*, June 1990, Institute of Psychiatry.

Lewis, G., Pelosi, A.J., Araya, R.C. and Dunn, G., (1992) Measuring psychiatric disorder in the community: a standardized assessment for use by lay interviewers, *Psychological Medicine*, **22**, 465-486

The CIS-R is an instrument used to measure neurotic psychopathology. More information about the CIS-R is included in Appendix A.

3   In Report 1, individuals were classified according to their most severe or primary disorder. The disorder hierarchy used to identify primary disorders is shown in Appendix A.

Summary of main findings

Background characteristics (Chapter 1)

- The survey classified 1,557 individuals, 16% of the sample, as having a neurotic disorder based on the frequency and severity of neurotic symptoms experienced in the seven days prior to interview.

- Just under half of these (48%) were adults classified as having mixed anxiety and depressive disorder and over a quarter (28%) had Generalised Anxiety Disorder (GAD). Fourteen per cent of adults with a neurotic disorder had depressive episode and 12% had phobias. Obsessive–Compulsive Disorder (OCD) was identified among 10% of adults with a neurotic disorder and 6% suffered from panic.

- Most (87%) of those with a neurotic disorder had only one disorder, 9% had two disorders and 4% had three or four disorders.

Physical complaints (Chapter 2)

The relationships described below show associations between neurotic disorders and physical complaints: no causal relationships should be assumed.

- 50% of adults with a neurotic disorder had a long-standing physical complaint compared with 30% of adults with no neurotic disorder.

- Musculo-skeletal complaints were the most common complaints and adults with a neurotic disorder were around twice as likely as those without disorder to have such complaints as others (23% and 11% respectively).

- Adults with neurosis were six times more likely than the sample without neurotic disorders to have genito-urinary complaints (6% compared with 1%).

- The proportions of adults with a physical complaint rose with increasing age, yet, at all ages, those with neurosis were more likely than those without a neurotic disorder to have a physical complaint.

- Compared with the group who had no neurotic disorders, both men and women with one neurotic disorder were around $1^1/_2$ times more likely to have a physical complaint, but those with two or more neurotic disorders were almost twice as likely to have such a complaint.

- The proportions of adults who were affected by a physical complaint did not vary widely in relation to type of neurotic disorder, ranging from 47% among those with GAD or phobia, to 55% of those with OCD.

- One in five adults who had a physical complaint also had a neurotic disorder, compared with one in ten of those with no physical complaint.

- Eight per cent of adults with a physical complaint reported significant symptoms of worry about their physical health compared with 3% of those with no physical complaints. Proportions were higher among those with a genito-urinary complaint (16%), and with neoplasms, musculo-skeletal or digestive system complaints (11%).

Treatment (Chapter 3)

- About 1 in 8 people with a neurotic disorder were currently having treatment. Among this group, two-thirds were taking medication and a half were having either therapy or counselling.

- Those classified as having two or more neurotic disorders were three times more likely to be receiving some form of treatment than those with one disorder (30% compared with 10%).

- The groups most likely to be receiving treatment were those classified as having a phobia (28%) or a depressive episode (25%); those least likely to be having some treatment were those with mixed anxiety and depressive disorder (9%).

- One factor increased the odds of getting all the treatments received: having more than one neurotic disorder.

- Compared with a reference group of 16–24 year olds, a greater proportion of those in older age groups were taking anxiolytics and hypnotics and this increased with the age of each group.

- About a third of those with a neurotic disorder who also reported having a long-standing, physical illness were taking medication for nervous system problems (31%). Drugs acting on cardiovascular, gastro-intestinal, respiratory, endocrine or musculo-skeletal systems were also taken by 10 to 15 percent of those with a neurotic disorder.

Use of services (Chapter 4)

- People with a neurotic disorder were about twice as likely as those without a disorder to consult a GP in the two weeks prior to interview (30% compared to 14%). The equivalent proportions who consulted a GP in the past year were: 79% and 62% for a physical complaint and 36% and 7% for a mental health problem.

- The largest increases in the odds of a GP

consultation for a mental health problem were associated with the presence of a neurotic disorder and of a physical illness. Among other factors, drug dependence was also associated with an increase in the odds of such a consultation.

- About 1 in 7 people (14%) with neurotic disorders had been a hospital in-patient during the year prior to interview, usually for a physical health problem.

- Half the adults with a neurotic disorder had visited a hospital, clinic or somewhere else for treatment or check-ups in the previous year, usually for a physical health problem and usually to a hospital out-patient department.

- A small minority of people with a neurotic disorder (3%) were currently attending a hospital or clinic for a mental health problem.

- A quarter of people with a neurotic disorder had not seen a doctor or other health professional about a mental problem in the past year, when they or others around them thought they should. This was usually because they either did not think anyone could help, or because they thought that they should be able to cope alone.

Adults with a psychotic disorder (Chapter 5)

- Adults with a psychotic disorder were equally represented among men and women. About half were aged 16–34 and the largest single proportion, 38%, were in the 25–34 age group.

- Fifty percent of adults with schizophrenia or bipolar affective disorder were married or cohabiting, 30% were single, and 20% were widowed, divorced or separated. Four in five of those who were living with a partner had at least one child.

- Compared with adults with no mental disorder, those with a psychotic disorder were about twice as likely to be unemployed or economically inactive, living in rented accommodation, living alone, or divorced or separated.

- Forty per cent of the group with a psychotic illness had a physical illness compared with 50% of those with a neurotic disorder and 30% of those without any disorder.

- About a half of all the adults identified as having a psychotic disorder were on medication or receiving counselling or therapy.

- In the 12 months prior to interview, 82% of those with a psychotic disorder had received some sort of service: two thirds had seen their GP for a 'mental or emotional problem', about a half had attended an out-patient clinic, and about one quarter had an in-patient stay.

Adults with suicidal thoughts
(Chapter 6)

Only those with significant depressive symptoms in terms of frequency, severity, or duration were also asked questions relating to depressive ideas including suicidal thoughts. Thus, people with suicidal thoughts who did not have significant depressive symptoms are not included in the analysis.

- Eighty informants, just less than 1% of the overall sample, said they had thoughts of killing themselves in the week prior to interview.

- About two thirds of those who had suicidal thoughts were women, and half were aged 16–34; 28% were aged 16–24. Half the sample were either living by themselves or without close relatives, or were lone parents.

- The group of adults with suicidal thoughts were about three times as likely as those with no mental disorder to be widowed, divorced or separated, and also three times more likely to be a lone parent or single person. They were also two and a half times more likely to be unemployed or economically inactive, and to be living in rented accommodation.

- All those with suicidal thoughts felt life was not worth living, 9 out of 10 had feelings of hopelessness, and at least 8 out of 10 felt 'not as good as others', the same proportion as those who blamed themselves when things went wrong.

- About a fifth of those who had thought about killing themselves in the week prior to interview were on antidepressants, the majority, two thirds, were taking tricyclic antidepressants.

- Among those with suicidal thoughts, about 6 out of 10 had seen their GP in the past year (about half of these in the past week), 5 out of 10 had been out-patients, about 3 in 10 in-patients and 1 in 10 had received a domiciliary visit.

- About 1 in 6 of the 80 adults identified by the survey as having suicidal thoughts were receiving counselling or therapy.

1 Characteristics of adults with neurotic disorders

1.1 Introduction

This chapter focuses on individuals who were identified as having various neurotic disorders and looks at the comorbidity of neurotic disorders. It shows the association between the neurotic disorders and CIS-R scores, and the distributions of key socio-demographic and socio-economic characteristics for those with each type of neurotic disorder and for those with no neurotic disorder. Finally, neurotic symptoms and the length of time since their onset are examined.

1.2 Neurotic disorders and their comorbidity

The survey classified 1,557 individuals, 16% of the sample, as having a neurotic disorder based on the frequency and severity of neurotic symptoms experienced in the seven days prior to interview. The numbers of adults who had each neurotic disorder are shown below. These figures form the bases used in subsequent tables.

The proportions of all adults who had each neurotic disorder are presented in *Table 1.1* alongside the proportions who had each disorder as their primary disorder. The hierarchy used to determine the primary disorder is shown in Appendix A. Mixed anxiety and depressive disorder could not be comorbid with any other neurotic disorder and affected 8% of all adults. Generalised anxiety disorder (GAD) affected 5% of all adults; for 3% of all adults it was their primary neurotic disorder, the other 2% of adults with GAD also had another, more severe neurotic disorder.

Just under half (48%) of adults with a neurotic disorder were classified as having mixed

The number of individuals with each neurotic disorder by sex

Disorder	Number of individuals with each disorder		
	Women	Men	All adults
Mixed anxiety and depressive disorder	485	265	750
Generalised Anxiety Disorder	251	188	439
Depressive episode	133	88	220
Phobia	122	58	180
Obsessive-Compulsive Disorder	100	57	157
Panic	50	43	93
Any neurotic disorder*	960	597	1557
No neurotic disorder	3948	4236	8184
*Base***	*4908*	*4833*	*9741*

* The column totals exceed the number of people with any neurotic disorder as some individuals had more than one neurotic disorder.

** These bases represent all adults who had a personal (ie non-proxy) interview, and who did not have a psychotic illness.

anxiety and depressive disorder while over a quarter (28%) had GAD. Fourteen per cent of adults with a neurotic disorder had depressive episode, either in mild, moderate or severe form; there was a roughly equal split between the three levels of severity. Phobias affected 12% of people with a neurotic disorder and were comprised of three types of phobia which were mutually exclusive: agoraphobia (5%), social phobia (4%) and specific isolated phobia (3%). Obsessive-Compulsive Disorder (OCD)

1

was identified among 10% of adults with a neurotic disorder and 6% suffered from panic. *(Table 1.2, Figure 1.1)*

Most (87%) of those with a neurotic disorder had only one disorder, 9% had two disorders and 4% had three or four disorders. More than two thirds of adults with OCD and at least half of those with depressive episode and phobia were identified as having comorbid neuroses. Other than mixed anxiety and depressive disorder which could not be comorbid, panic and GAD were most likely to be found in isolation; over two thirds of adults with these disorders had just one neurotic disorder. *(Table 1.3)*

The comorbidity between individual disorders is shown in Table 1.4. Of all adults with OCD, the most comorbid disorder, 40% also had GAD, 33% had depressive episode, 26% had phobia and 4% had panic disorder. Over a third of adults with depressive episode also suffered from GAD. Sex differences in

patterns of comorbidity between individual neurotic disorders were not marked. *(Table 1.4)*

1.3 CIS-R scores and neurotic disorders

Forty five per cent of those with a neurotic disorder had CIS-R scores between 12-17 and a further 45% had scores of 18 or more. Scores of the highest order were most common among adults with depressive episode, OCD and phobia with over 70% scoring 18 or more on the CIS-R. While only 10% of all adults with a neurotic disorder had CIS-R scores below 12, the figures were notably higher among those with Generalised Anxiety Disorder (23%) and panic disorder (22%).
(Table 1.5, Figure 1.2)

Ninety per cent of those with 2 or more neurotic disorders had CIS-R scores of 18 or more, as did 38% of those with one neurotic disorder. *(Table 1.6)*

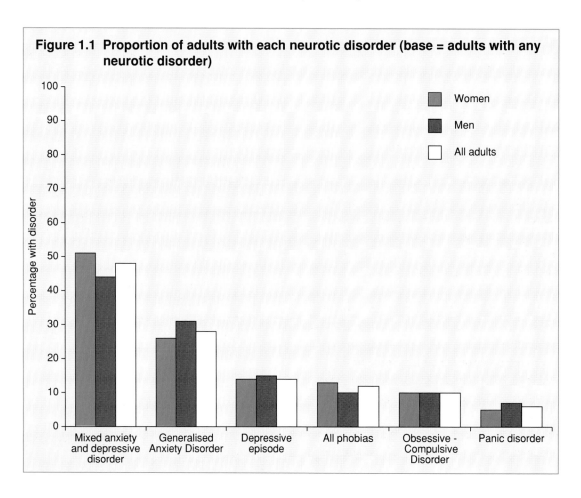

Figure 1.1 Proportion of adults with each neurotic disorder (base = adults with any neurotic disorder)

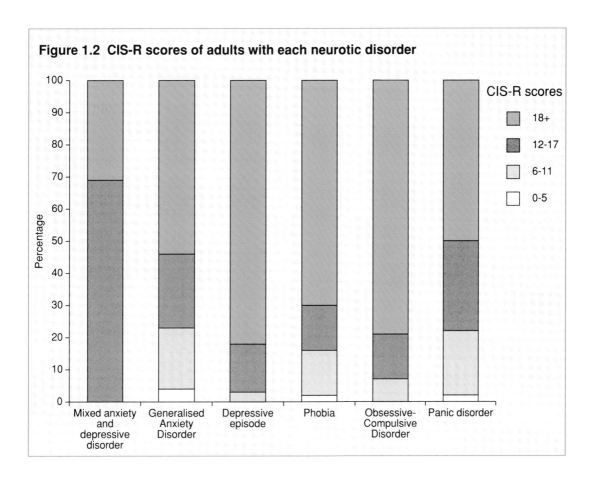

Figure 1.2 CIS-R scores of adults with each neurotic disorder

1.4 Characteristics of those with neurotic disorders

This section compares those identified as having a neurotic disorder with those from the remainder of the sample in terms of various characteristics. The major socio-demographic and socio-economic differences identified between these groups were sex, employment status, housing tenure and the type of family unit into which survey respondents were classified. Variations were also found in marital status and educational qualifications.

The data discussed in this section are found in Tables 1.7 to 1.10. The following are the most striking, significant findings, arranged according to the order of the tables. Some of the variables in the tables are inter-related; however this chapter does not consider the strength of independent effects; Report 1 (Chapter 6) did show the odds ratios of socio-demographic and socio-economic correlates in relation to psychiatric morbidity.

Compared with those with no neurotic disorder, those with a neurotic disorder were...

more likely to be:
- women (62% compared with 38%)
- widowed, divorced or separated (15% compared with 9%)
- lone parents (10% compared with 5%)
- living in one-person family units (18% compared with 13%)
- people with no educational qualifications (35% compared with 28%)
- unemployed or economically inactive (44% compared with 29%)
- living in rented accommodation (39% compared with 25%)
- living in urban areas (72% compared with 65%)

less likely to be:
- married (53% compared with 61%)
- people with GCE A-levels or higher educational qualifications (30% compared with 35%)

1.5 Characteristics of those with each neurotic disorder

Although many of the characteristics of adults with any neurotic disorder were common to those with each of the named disorders, some characteristics are particularly associated with individual disorders. The following findings are drawn from Tables 1.7 to 1.10 and again are presented in the table order, rather than in order of significance. As the bases for some of the disorders were very small, some apparent differences did not reach statistical significance; some of these findings are included in the commentary, but are marked (NS).

i) Generalised Anxiety Disorder

Compared with adults with no neurotic disorder, those with GAD were...

more likely to be:
- women (57% compared with 48%)
- aged 35-64 (71% compared with 56%)
- women aged 45-64 (50% compared with 35%)
- men aged 35-54 (54% compared with 39%)
- widowed (10% compared with 5%)
- people with no educational qualifications (43% compared with 28%)
- economically inactive or unemployed 36% and 15% (compared with 21% and 8%)
- renting their home from a Housing Association or Local Authority (31% compared with 16%)
- urban dwellers (74% compared with 65%)

less likely to be:
- women aged 16-34 (30% compared with 44%)
- men aged 16-24 (7% compared with 20%)
- single (14% compared with 20%)

ii) Depressive episode

Compared with adults with no neurotic disorder, those with depressive episode were...

more likely to be:
- women (60% compared with 48%)
- divorced or separated (17% compared with 7%)
- living in one-person family units (20% compared with 13%)
- lone parents (13% compared with 5%)
- people with no educational qualifications (40% compared with 28%)
- economically inactive (40% compared with 21%)
- urban dwellers (74% compared with 65%)

less likely to be:
- married (46% compared with 61%)
- living in couples without children (18% compared with 27%)
- in Social Classes I or II (18% compared with 34%)

iii) Phobia

Compared with adults with no neurotic disorder, those with phobia were...

more likely to be:
- women (68% compared with 48%)
- aged 16-24 (28% compared with 19%) - social phobia was associated with age far more than agoraphobia or specific isolated phobia; 41% of those with social phobia were aged 16-24 (table not shown)
- non-white (9% compared with 5%, NS)
- lone parents (14% compared with 5%)
- people with no educational qualifications (38% compared with 28%)
- economically inactive (48% compared with 21%)
- unemployed (18% compared with 8%)
- living in rented accommodation (45% compared with 25%)

less likely to be:
- married (41% compared with 61%)
- living in a couple with children (29% compared with 40%)
- people with GCE A-levels or higher qualifications (20% compared with 35%)
- in Social Class I or II (19% compared with 34%)
- rural dwellers (5% compared with 11%)

iv) Obsessive-Compulsive Disorder

Compared with adults with no neurotic disorder, those with Obsessive-Compulsive Disorder were...

more likely to be:
- women (64% compared with 48%)
- aged 16-24 (24% compared with 19%, NS)
- divorced (11% compared with 5%)
- people living in one-person family units (22% compared with 13%)
- lone parents (12% compared with 5%)
- people with no educational qualifications (39% compared with 28%)
- living in accommodation rented from a Housing Association or Local Authority (28% compared with 16%)
- living in Wales (11% compared with 5%, NS)

less likely to be:
- married (50% compared with 61%)
- living in a couple with children (29% compared with 40%)
- people with GCE A-levels or higher qualifications (23% compared with 35%)
- working (55% compared with 71%)

v) Panic disorder

Compared with adults with no neurotic disorder, those with panic disorder were...

more likely to be:
- men aged 45-54 or 16-24 (27% and 26% compared with 19% and 20%, NS)
- widowed women (13% compared with 3%)

- people with no educational qualifications (42% compared with 28%)
- living in accommodation rented from a Housing Association or Local Authority (37% compared with 16%)

less likely to be:
- women living in couples without children (13% compared with 29%)
- living in Wales (no cases compared with 5%)

vi) Mixed anxiety and depressive disorder

Since the largest proportion of adults with any neurotic disorder were classified as having mixed anxiety and depressive disorder, the characteristics of this group were generally similar to those of the above, as described in section 1.4. However, for some characteristics the relationships for mixed anxiety and depression were weaker than for other, specific, neurotic disorders. for example, 60% of those with mixed anxiety and depression were in employment; this represents a higher proportion than for any of the other neurotic disorders and is almost as high as those with no disorder (71%). The distribution of educational qualifications for those with mixed anxiety and depressive disorder was no different from that for adults with no neurotic disorder. *(Tables 1.7 to 1.9)*

1.6 Neurotic symptoms and their effects

As described in Appendix A, diagnoses of neurotic disorders were based on the informant's experiences of 14 symptoms covered by the CIS-R in the previous 7 days. Table 1.10 shows the proportion of people with each disorder who had significant symptoms. Although some symptoms affected a sizeable proportion of adults with no neurotic disorder, particularly fatigue, sleep problems and irritability (affecting 14%-17%), not surprisingly all of the symptoms were far more prevalent among those with neurotic disorders. Fatigue and worry were the most prevalent symptoms among those with a neurotic disorder, affecting 77% and 67% respectively.

Other than for OCD and mixed anxiety and depressive disorder, for each disorder there was a dominant diagnostic symptom which must have been present in order for that disorder to be diagnosed. For example, a diagnosis of depressive episode required the presence of depression symptoms. Such symptoms will of course have been present for 100% of cases of these disorders. OCD required *either* significant obsessive *or* compulsive symptoms and among those with OCD, 92% had obsessions and 48% had compulsions. Mixed anxiety and depressive disorder did not require any significant symptoms to be present, and four out of five people classified as having mixed anxiety and depressive disorder suffered from fatigue with two thirds experiencing sleep problems. *(Table 1.10)*

For each symptom that was present in the previous seven days respondents were asked how long they had experienced the feelings they had described. Table 1.11 presents the main diagnostic symptom(s) associated with each neurotic disorder. For example, for GAD the table shows how long the informants experienced anxiety and for OCD it shows firstly how long they experienced obsessions and secondly, how long they experienced compulsions. Mixed anxiety and depressive disorder is not shown here, as classification of this disorder was not based on any particular symptom. Many of the adults identified as having a neurotic disorder had been affected by them for a considerable length of time. For example, 61% of those with GAD had experienced anxiety for over two years, and 35% of those with severe depressive episode had experienced symptoms of depression for over one year. *(Table 1.11)*

Respondents who had at least one significant neurotic symptom were asked whether the way they had been feeling during the past week had actually stopped them from getting on with things they used to do or would like to do, or whether it had not stopped activities, but had made them more difficult. Over half (54%) the adults with neurosis reported that the way they had been feeling had stopped them from getting on with things, compared with 16% of symptomatic adults who failed the criteria of full neurotic disorder. However, there was no significant difference between these two groups in the proportions who reported that their activities had merely been made more difficult (31% and 27% respectively). All of those with phobia or OCD, and 91% of those with depressive episode said that the way they had been feeling during the past week had actually stopped them from getting on with things. *(Table 1.12)*

Table 1.1   Proportion of all adults with each disorder, and the primary disorder* distribution by sex

All adults

Disorder	Individuals with each disorder			Individuals with primary disorder*		
	Women	Men	All adults	Women	Men	All adults
	Percentage with disorder **			%	%	%
Mixed anxiety and depressive disorder	10	5	8	10	5	8
Generalised Anxiety Disorder	5	4	5	3	3	3
Depressive episode	3	2	2	2	2	2
Phobia	2	1	2	1	1	1
Obsessive-Compulsive Disorder	2	1	2	1	1	1
Panic	1	1	1	1	1	1
No disorder	80	88	84	80	88	84
Base	*4908*	*4833*	*9741*	*4908*	*4833*	*9741*

*   Individuals were classified according to their most severe neurotic disorder; primary disorder

** The percentages in these columns exceed 100% as some individuals had more than one neurotic disorder

Table 1.2   Percentage of people with each disorder by sex

All respondents with a neurotic disorder

Disorder	Women	Men	All adults
	Percentage with each disorder		
Mixed anxiety and depressive disorder	51	44	48
Generalised Anxiety Disorder	26	31	28
Depressive episode			
mild	5	6	6
moderate	4	3	4
severe	5	5	5
All	14	15	14
Phobia			
agoraphobia	5	3	5
social	4	5	4
specific isolated	4	2	3
All	13	10	12
Obsessive-Compulsive Disorder	10	10	10
Panic	5	7	6
Base	*960*	*597*	*1557*

Table 1.3   Number of neurotic disorders by disorder and sex

Respondents who had a neurotic disorder

Number of neurotic disorders	Mixed anxiety and depressive disorder	Generalised Anxiety Disorder		Depressive episode		Phobia		Obsessive-Compulsive Disorder		Panic disorder		Any neurotic disorder	
	%	%		%		%		%		%		%	
Women													
1	100	65		40		50		33		70		86	
2	-	20		34		28		34		18		9	
3	-	12	35	20	60	15	50	25	67	11	30	4	14
4	-	3		6		6		8		1		1	
Base	*485*	*251*		*133*		*122*		*100*		*50*		*960*	
Men													
1	100	70		43		51		41		71		87	
2	-	21		41		30		32		19		10	
3	-	7	30	12	57	14	49	20	59	7	29	3	13
4	-	2		4		4		6		2		1	
Base	*265*	*188*		*88*		*58*		*57*		*43*		*597*	
All adults													
1	100	67		41		51		36		70		87	
2	-	20		37		29		33		19		9	
3	-	10	33	17	59	15	49	24	64	9	30	3	13
4	-	3		5		6		7		2		1	
Base	*750*	*439*		*220*		*180*		*157*		*93*		*1557*	

Table 1.4 Comorbidity among neurotic disorders by sex

Respondents who had a neurotic disorder

Comorbid disorder	Mixed anxiety and depressive disorder	Generalised Anxiety Disorder	Depressive episode	Phobia	Obsessive-Compulsive Disorder	Panic disorder	Any neurotic disorder
	Percentage with each comorbid disorder						
Women							
Mixed anxiety and depressive disorder	*	-	-	-	-	-	51
Generalised Anxiety Disorder	-	*	36	30	40	20	26
Depressive episode	-	19	*	24	37	16	14
Phobia	-	15	22	*	27	-	13
Obsessive-Compulsive Disorder	-	16	28	22	*	8	10
Panic	-	4	6	-	4	*	5
Base	*485*	*251*	*133*	*122*	*100*	*50*	*960*
Men							
Mixed anxiety and depressive disorder	*	-	-	-	-	-	44
Generalised Anxiety Disorder	-	*	37	25	38	16	31
Depressive episode	-	17	*	24	25	17	15
Phobia	-	8	16	*	23	-	10
Obsessive-Compulsive Disorder	-	12	16	23	*	7	10
Panic	-	4	8	-	5	*	7
Base	*265*	*188*	*88*	*58*	*57*	*43*	*597*
All adults							
Mixed anxiety and depressive disorder	*	-	-	-	-	-	48
Generalised Anxiety Disorder	-	*	36	28	40	18	28
Depressive episode	-	18	*	24	33	16	14
Phobia	-	12	20	*	26	-	12
Obsessive-Compulsive Disorder	-	14	23	23	*	8	10
Panic	-	4	7	-	4	*	6
Base	*750*	*439*	*220*	*180*	*157*	*93*	*1557*

Table 1.5 The CIS-R scores of those with different neurotic disorders

All adults

CIS-R score	Mixed anxiety and depressive disorder	Generalised Anxiety Disorder	Depressive episode	Phobia	Obsessive-Compulsive Disorder	Panic disorder	Any neurotic disorder	No neurotic disorder
	%	%	%	%	%	%	%	%
0-5	-	4	-	2	-	2	1	79
6-11	-	19	3	14	7	20	9	21
0-11	**-**	**22**	**3**	**16**	**7**	**22**	**10**	**100**
12-17	69	23	15	14	14	28	45	-
18+	31	55	82	70	79	50	45	-
12 +	**100**	**78**	**97**	**84**	**93**	**78**	**90**	**-**
Base	*750*	*439*	*220*	*180*	*157*	*93*	*1557*	*8184*

Table 1.6 CIS-R scores by the number of neurotic disorders

All adults

CIS-R score	Number of neurotic disorders			
	0	1	2 or more	All
	%	%	%	%
0-5	79	2	-	66
6-11	21	10	1	19
0-11	**100**	**12**	**1**	**86**
12-17	-	51	9	7
18+	-	38	90	7
12+	**-**	**88**	**99**	**14**
Base	*6456*	*1890*	*702*	*9741*

Table 1.7   Age, ethnicity, marital status and family unit type by neurotic disorder and sex

	Mixed anxiety and depressive disorder	Generalised Anxiety Disorder	Depressive episode	All phobias	Obsessive-Compulsive Disorder	Panic disorder	Any neurotic disorder	No neurotic disorder
	%	%	%	%	%	%	%	%
Women								
Age								
16-24	19	12	22	31	26	15	19	19
25-34	28	18	30	24	20	29	25	25
35-44	25	20	20	17	24	20	23	21
45-54	19	28	21	16	18	21	21	18
55-64	8	22	7	11	12	15	12	17
Ethnicity								
White	92	97	93	93	95	95	94	95
West Indian or African	2	1	-	1	-	1	2	2
Asian or Oriental	5	2	5	3	3	4	4	3
Other	1	1	1	2	2	-	1	1
Marital status								
Married	52	57	43	39	46	53	52	62
Cohabiting	10	9	8	12	5	4	9	7
Single	21	14	26	33	27	18	21	20
Widowed	3	6	5	3	4	13	5	3
Divorced	10	10	11	10	13	9	10	5
Separated	3	3	6	4	6	2	4	2
Family unit type								
Couple, no children	21	28	15	21	25	13	22	29
Couple and child(ren)	41	38	36	30	25	45	39	40
Lone parent and child(ren)	15	13	20	19	19	21	15	9
One person only	16	14	18	12	20	13	16	11
Adult with parents	5	4	6	17	7	8	7	9
Adult with one parent	2	2	5	1	4	-	2	2
Base	*485*	*251*	*133*	*122*	*100*	*50*	*960*	*3948*

11

Table 1.7 Age, ethnicity, marital status and family unit type by neurotic disorder and sex - *continued*

	Mixed anxiety and depressive disorder	Generalised Anxiety Disorder	Depressive episode	All phobias	Obsessive-Compulsive Disorder	Panic disorder	Any neurotic disorder	No neurotic disorder
Men	%	%	%	%	%	%	%	%
Age								
16-24	16	7	19	21	19	26	16	20
25-34	30	23	16	27	21	23	26	25
35-44	22	28	20	15	24	14	23	20
45-54	14	26	26	26	24	27	19	19
55-64	17	16	18	12	12	10	16	16
Ethnicity								
White	94	95	94	88	98	99	94	94
West Indian or African	2	2	2	1	–	1	2	1
Asian or Oriental	4	1	4	8	–	–	3	3
Other	1	2	1	4	2	–	1	1
Marital status								
Married	56	61	51	46	57	54	56	60
Cohabiting	8	3	4	10	4	3	6	7
Single	28	25	26	25	29	35	28	28
Widowed	2	1	3	2	–	2	1	1
Divorced	5	6	9	11	7	5	6	4
Separated	2	4	7	6	3	1	3	1
Family unit type								
Couple, no children	23	21	22	28	24	28	23	26
Couple and child(ren)	41	43	32	27	36	28	39	41
Lone parent and child(ren)	2	2	2	3	2	5	2	1
One person only	20	23	25	27	26	13	21	14
Adult with parents	8	6	16	11	10	16	10	14
Adult with one parent	6	4	2	4	3	10	5	4
Base	*265*	*188*	*88*	*58*	*57*	*43*	*597*	*4236*

Table 1.7 Age, ethnicity, marital status and family unit type by neurotic disorder and sex - *continued*

	Mixed anxiety and depressive disorder	Generalised Anxiety Disorder	Depressive episode	All phobias	Obsessive-Compulsive Disorder	Panic disorder	Any neurotic disorder	No neurotic disorder
All adults	%	%	%	%	%	%	%	%
Sex								
Women	65	57	60	68	64	54	62	48
Men	35	43	40	32	37	46	38	52
Age								
16-24	18	10	21	28	24	20	18	19
25-34	29	20	25	25	20	26	26	25
35-44	24	23	20	16	24	18	23	21
45-54	17	28	23	19	20	24	20	19
55-64	12	20	11	12	12	12	14	16
Ethnicity								
White	93	96	93	91	96	97	94	95
West Indian or African	2	1	1	1	-	1	2	2
Asian or Oriental	4	1	5	5	2	2	4	3
Other	1	1	1	3	2	-	1	1
Marital status								
Married	53	59	46	41	50	53	53	61
Cohabiting	9	7	6	11	5	4	8	7
Single	24	19	26	30	28	26	24	24
Widowed	3	6	5	3	4	13	5	3
Divorced	8	8	10	10	11	7	8	5
Separated	3	3	7	4	4	2	3	2
Family unit type								
Couple, no children	22	25	18	23	25	20	22	27
Couple and child(ren)	41	40	35	29	29	37	39	40
Lone parent and child(ren)	10	9	13	14	12	13	10	5
One person only	18	18	20	17	22	13	18	13
Adult with parents	6	5	10	15	8	12	8	12
Adult with one parent	3	3	4	2	4	4	3	3
Base	*750*	*439*	*220*	*180*	*157*	*93*	*1557*	*8184*

Table 1.8   Educational qualifications, social class, employment status and tenure by neurotic disorder and sex

	Mixed anxiety and depressive disorder	Generalised Anxiety Disorder	Depressive episode	All phobias	Obsessive-Compulsive Disorder	Panic disorder	Any neurotic disorder	No neurotic disorder
Women	%	%	%	%	%	%	%	%
Qualifications								
A level or higher	29	20	26	19	19	22	25	28
GCSE/O level	26	22	22	30	28	25	26	28
Other	14	8	12	11	15	10	12	12
None	31	51	41	40	39	43	38	32
Social class								
I	6	3	4	1	6	2	5	6
II	25	20	13	13	18	24	21	28
IIIN	18	18	21	23	19	23	19	17
IIIM	26	27	27	24	25	31	26	26
IV	18	19	24	23	15	12	19	15
V	5	10	7	7	11	6	6	5
Armed forces	1	-	-	1	2	3	1	1
Never worked	1	2	3	7	4	-	2	2
Employment status								
Working full time	33	27	17	14	26	33	29	36
Working part time	25	19	24	16	21	24	24	29
Unemployed	11	10	14	15	12	5	11	4
Economically inactive	30	44	46	55	41	37	36	30
Tenure								
Owned outright	11	15	14	11	12	19	13	18
Owned with mortgage	50	44	44	45	50	45	49	55
Rented from HA or LA	29	33	31	34	28	31	18	29
Rented from other source	10	8	11	9	10	5	9	8
Base	*485*	*251*	*133*	*122*	*100*	*50*	*960*	*3948*

Table 1.8   **Educational qualifications, social class, employment status and tenure by neurotic disorder and sex**- *continued*

	Mixed anxiety and depressive disorder	Generalised Anxiety Disorder	Depressive episode	All phobias	Obsessive-Compulsive Disorder	Panic disorder	Any neurotic disorder	No neurotic disorder
Men	%	%	%	%	%	%	%	%
Qualifications								
A level or higher	42	33	21	22	30	40	37	41
GCSE/O level	27	20	28	31	21	14	24	24
Other	6	13	13	12	11	7	9	10
None	25	34	39	35	38	40	30	25
Social class								
I	4	5	2	2	-	-	4	8
II	28	26	17	26	37	31	28	25
IIIN	15	16	18	12	7	6	14	12
IIIM	33	30	35	30	34	25	32	31
IV	11	18	13	21	16	15	14	15
V	5	3	13	6	5	16	6	5
Armed forces	1	-	-	-	-	-	-	1
Never worked	2	1	2	4	2	7	2	2
Employment status								
Working full time	57	46	45	38	51	49	52	71
Working part time	6	7	5	5	3	3	6	6
Unemployed	17	22	20	24	20	23	20	11
Economically inactive	20	25	30	33	27	24	22	13
Tenure								
Owned outright	12	15	12	10	18	11	12	16
Owned with mortgage	53	44	40	42	42	30	48	60
Rented from HA or LA	22	28	38	42	29	44	27	15
Rented from other source	13	13	10	6	11	14	13	10
Base	*265*	*188*	*88*	*58*	*57*	*43*	*597*	*4236*

15

Table 1.8   Educational qualifications, social class, employment status and tenure by neurotic disorder and sex - *continued*

	Mixed anxiety and depressive disorder	Generalised Anxiety Disorder	Depressive episode	All phobias	Obsessive-Compulsive Disorder	Panic disorder	Any neurotic disorder	No neurotic disorder
All adults	%	%	%	%	%	%	%	%
Qualifications								
A level or higher	33	25	24	20	23	30	30	35
GCSE/O level	26	21	24	30	25	20	25	26
Other	11	10	12	11	13	9	11	11
None	29	43	40	38	39	42	35	28
Social class								
I	5	4	3	1	4	1	4	7
II	26	22	15	18	25	27	24	27
IIIN	17	17	20	19	15	15	17	15
IIIM	29	29	30	26	28	28	28	28
IV	15	19	20	22	15	13	17	15
V	5	7	10	7	9	11	6	5
Armed forces	1	-	-	1	2	1	1	1
Never worked	2	1	3	6	3	3	2	2
Employment status								
Working full time	42	35	28	22	35	41	38	54
Working part time	18	14	16	12	14	14	17	17
Unemployed	14	15	16	18	15	13	14	8
Economically inactive	26	36	40	48	36	31	30	21
Tenure								
Owned outright	11	15	13	10	14	16	13	17
Owned with mortgage	51	44	42	44	47	38	48	58
Rented from HA or LA	27	31	34	37	28	37	28	16
Rented from other source	11	10	11	8	10	9	11	9
Base	*750*	*439*	*220*	*180*	*157*	*93*	*1557*	*8184*

Table 1.9 Region, country and locality by neurotic disorder and sex

	Mixed anxiety and depressive disorder	Generalised Anxiety Disorder	Depressive episode	All phobias	Obsessive-Compulsive Disorder	Panic disorder	Any neurotic disorder	No neurotic disorder
Women	%	%	%	%	%	%	%	%
Regional Health Authority								
Northern	7	8	5	8	5	2	7	6
Yorkshire	9	10	10	5	7	11	9	8
Trent	7	7	6	8	6	4	7	11
East Anglia	4	5	8	4	5	4	5	5
NW Thames	8	7	6	5	7	10	7	7
NE Thames	11	9	10	8	11	13	10	6
SE Thames	9	11	10	8	7	5	9	8
SW Thames	8	2	4	10	6	1	6	6
Wessex	4	5	4	10	11	8	5	7
Oxford	4	5	2	8	1	5	4	6
South Western	5	3	6	3	4	5	4	6
West Midlands	10	11	14	10	16	13	11	10
Mersey	8	9	8	7	7	2	7	5
North Western	7	7	7	6	8	16	8	8
Base	*426*	*219*	*117*	*108*	*81*	*44*	*840*	*3457*
Country								
England	88	87	88	88	81	87	88	88
Scotland	7	5	8	5	8	13	7	7
Wales	6	7	4	7	11	–	6	5
Locality								
Urban	73	75	76	74	67	70	73	64
Semi-rural	19	18	17	20	25	12	19	25
Rural	8	7	7	6	8	18	8	11
Base	*485*	*251*	*133*	*122*	*100*	*50*	*960*	*3948*

Table 1.9 Region, country and locality by neurotic disorder and sex - *continued*

	Mixed anxiety and depressive disorder	Generalised Anxiety Disorder	Depressive episode	All phobias	Obsessive-Compulsive Disorder	Panic disorder	Any neurotic disorder	No neurotic disorder
Men	%	%	%	%	%	%	%	%
Regional Health Authority								
Northern	7	8	5	1	5	4	7	6
Yorkshire	3	11	10	7	14	13	6	8
Trent	14	11	8	12	8	12	13	12
East Anglia	3	2	2	–	–	3	2	4
NW Thames	6	8	7	13	12	5	7	8
NE Thames	6	9	11	7	6	14	8	8
SE Thames	8	8	5	8	14	-	8	8
SW Thames	6	8	4	11	2	6	7	6
Wessex	8	4	8	6	9	5	6	7
Oxford	6	5	6	8	5	1	6	6
South Western	7	3	3	5	1	3	5	6
West Midlands	15	9	11	6	12	19	12	10
Mersey	4	9	6	7	9	–	6	4
North Western	7	5	13	9	2	16	7	8
Base	*240*	*165*	*74*	*50*	*44*	*42*	*529*	*3746*
Country								
England	90	88	85	86	78	97	89	88
Scotland	7	6	6	10	13	3	6	6
Wales	3	6	10	4	10	–	5	5
Locality								
Urban	68	73	72	82	77	69	71	65
Semi-urban	24	20	23	15	21	23	22	24
Rural	8	7	5	3	2	8	7	11
Base	*265*	*188*	*88*	*58*	*57*	*43*	*597*	*4236*

Table 1.9 Region, country and locality by neurotic disorder and sex - *continued*

	Mixed anxiety and depressive disorder	Generalised Anxiety Disorder	Depressive episode	All phobias	Obsessive-Compulsive Disorder	Panic disorder	Any neurotic disorder	No neurotic disorder
All adults	%	%	%	%	%	%	%	%
Regional Health Authority								
Northern	7	8	5	6	5	3	7	6
Yorkshire	7	10	10	5	10	12	8	8
Trent	9	9	7	9	6	8	9	11
East Anglia	4	4	6	2	3	3	4	4
NW Thames	7	7	6	8	9	8	7	8
NE Thames	9	9	10	8	9	13	9	7
SE Thames	9	10	8	8	10	2	9	8
SW Thames	7	5	4	10	4	4	7	6
Wessex	5	4	6	9	10	7	5	7
Oxford	5	5	4	8	2	3	5	6
South Western	6	3	5	4	3	4	5	6
West Midlands	12	10	12	9	15	16	11	10
Mersey	6	9	7	7	8	1	7	5
North Western	7	6	9	7	6	16	8	8
Base	*666*	*385*	*191*	*158*	*126*	*85*	*1369*	*7203*
Country								
England	89	88	87	88	80	92	88	88
Scotland	7	6	7	6	10	8	7	7
Wales	5	7	6	6	11	-	5	5
Locality								
Urban	71	74	74	77	71	70	72	65
Semi-urban	21	19	19	18	24	17	20	24
Rural	78	7	6	5	6	13	7	11
Base	*750*	*439*	*220*	*180*	*157*	*93*	*1557*	*8184*

Table 1.10   The prevalence of symptoms measured on the CIS-R by neurotic disorder

All adults

Symptom	Mixed anxiety and depressive disorder	General-ised Anxiety Disorder	Depressive episode	Phobia	Obsessive-Compulsive Disorder	Panic disorder	Any neurotic disorder	No neurotic disorder	More than one disorder
	Percentage of adults experiencing symptom								
Fatigue	81	72	86	76	77	74	77	17	88
Sleep problems	67	60	75	63	63	54	63	17	74
Irritability	61	61	72	70	62	68	61	14	75
Worry	65	74	81	69	83	58	67	11	88
Depression	35	42	100	53	60	35	43	3	76
Depressive ideas	42	44	81	56	66	39	46	2	73
Anxiety	24	100	62	50	59	47	47	2	85
Obsessions	33	34	43	40	92	26	35	4	61
Concentration & forgetfulness	33	38	57	54	43	34	36	2	58
Somatic symptoms	30	32	35	28	32	32	29	3	38
Compulsions	16	20	21	39	48	28	20	4	36
Phobias	12	23	30	100	36	-	22	2	51
Worry-physical health	16	24	31	31	29	17	19	2	33
Panic	4	21	26	33	23	100	15	0	43
Base	*750*	*439*	*220*	*180*	*157*	*93*	*1557*	*8184*	*209*

Table 1.11   How long people had been experiencing the symptoms involved in the diagnosis of neurotic disorders

All adults with neurotic disorder other than mixed anxiety and depressive disorder

Time for which symptom experienced	Generalised Anxiety Disorder & anxiety	Mild depressive episode & depression	Moderate depressive episode & depression	Severe depressive episode & depression	Agora-phobia & phobia	Social phobia & phobia	Specific isolated phobia & phobia	Obsessive-Compulsive Disorder & obsessions	Obsessive-Compulsive Disorder & compulsions	Panic disorder & panic
	%	%	%	%	%	%	%	%	%	%
Less than 2 weeks	-	-	-	12	2	11	6	3	11	16
2 weeks - less than 6 months	-	31	36	27	24	27	11	30	27	17
6 months - less than 1 year	22	23	22	26	8	6	7	14	10	9
1 year - less than 2 years	17	11	11	11	15	11	2	16	20	13
2 years or more	61	35	32	24	52	46	73	37	33	46
Base	*439*	*86*	*56*	*79*	*71*	*61*	*47*	*146*	*88*	*93*

Table 1.12 Severity of limiting effects of symptoms by neurotic disorder

Adults who had any significant symptom

Severity of limiting effects	Mixed anxiety and depressive disorder	Generalised Anxiety Disorder	Depressive episode	Phobia	Obsessive-Compulsive Disorder	Panic disorder	Any neurotic disorder	No neurotic disorder
	Percentage for whom the way they were feeling stopped activities or made them more difficult							
Women								
stopped activities	38	47	89	100	100	44	51	15
activities more difficult	44	27	11	-	-	38	32	27
Base	*485*	*251*	*133*	*122*	*100*	*50*	*960*	*2122*
Men								
stopped activities	43	57	95	100	100	58	58	17
activities more difficult	37	28	5	-	-	35	28	27
Base	*265*	*188*	*88*	*58*	*57*	*43*	*597*	*1654*
All adults								
stopped activities	40	51	91	100	100	50	54	16
activities more difficult	42	27	9	-	-	37	31	27
Base	*750*	*439*	*220*	*180*	*157*	*93*	*1557*	*3776*

2 Neurotic disorders and physical complaints

2.1 Introduction

This chapter looks at neurotic disorders and chronic physical illness, including disability and infirmity, and addresses the question of the association between them: to what extent do physical complaints co-occur with neurotic disorders? Multiple logistic regression models were also used to explore the associations between neurotic disorder and physical complaints, controlling for various socio-demographic and socio-economic characteristics.

We also consider whether adults with physical complaints differ from others in the extent to which they worry about their physical health, as measured by the CIS–R.

Although data were collected on the time of onset of neurotic symptoms and of physical complaints, it is not possible to identify causal relationships between neurotic disorder and physical complaints for the following reasons:

- symptom onset data cannot be directly related to the onset of a specific neurotic disorder

- onset data are difficult to interpret due to the episodic nature and varying severity of neurotic symptoms and physical complaints

- the unreliability of onset data due to memory effects.

Thus, this chapter explores associations between neurotic disorders and physical illness: no causal relationships should be assumed.

Measurement and classification of chronic physical complaints

Information was collected from all respondents about self-reported chronic ill-health using the following question:

> "Do you have any long-standing illness, disability or infirmity? By long-standing I mean something that has troubled you over a period of time or that is likely to affect you over a period of time?"

This question has been widely used in national surveys, taken from the General Household Survey.[1]

Those who answered 'Yes', were then asked:

> "What is the matter with you?"

Responses were coded according to the site or system of the body that was affected, using a classification system that roughly corresponded to the chapter headings of the International Classification of Diseases (ICD–10):[2]

Physical complaints of the:
- Musculo-skeletal system and connective tissue
- Respiratory system
- Heart and circulatory system
- Digestive system
- Nervous system and sense organs
- Endocrine, nutritional and metabolic diseases and immunity disorders
- Genito-urinary system
- Skin and sub-cutaneous tissue
- Ear and mastoid process
- Eye and adnexa
- Neoplasms (including benign and non-specific growths or lumps)
- Infectious and parasitic diseases

Because of the difficulty in distinguishing between malignant and non-malignant conditions from the respondents' self-report, 'neoplasms' included benign and non-specific growths or lumps.

2.2 Neurotic disorder and physical complaints

Overall, 33% of adults had a physical complaint, most commonly a musculo-skeletal complaint (13%). Estimates of the prevalence of physical complaints compare well with those of the 1989 General Household Survey which asked the same questions in a general population sample of 15,734 adults aged 16 to 64, and used the same classification system. Estimates of the proportions of adults with each physical complaint differed by no more than a percentage point, although in this survey the 13% suffering from musculo-skeletal complaints was significantly different from the GHS estimate of 11%. *(Table 2.1)*

Having a neurotic disorder had a marked negative association with physical well-being; 50% of adults with neurosis were affected by physical complaints compared with 30% of adults with no disorder.

Adults with neurosis were around twice as likely to suffer musculo-skeletal complaints as other adults (23% and 11% respectively). There was a six-fold difference in the proportions of adults suffering from genito-urinary complaints; affecting 6% of neurotic adults and 1% of those with no disorder. Neurotic adults were also more likely than others to be affected by complaints of the respiratory, heart and circulatory, digestive, or nervous system. *(Table 2.1, Figure 2.1)*

Age

As expected, the likelihood of having a physical complaint increased with age, but at all ages, adults with neurosis were much more likely to have a physical complaint than those who did not have neurosis.

Adults aged between 25 and 54 who had a neurotic disorder were around twice as likely to have a physical complaint compared with their counterparts who did not have a neurotic disorder. The same relationship was found for younger women, aged 16 to 24. *(Table 2.2, Figure 2.2)*

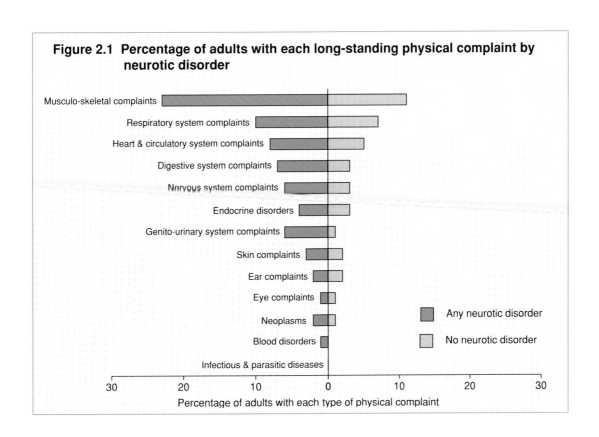

Figure 2.1 **Percentage of adults with each long-standing physical complaint by neurotic disorder**

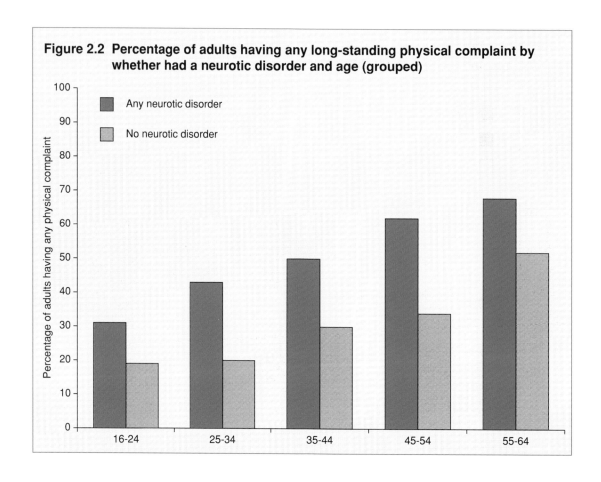

Figure 2.2 Percentage of adults having any long-standing physical complaint by whether had a neurotic disorder and age (grouped)

2.3 The number of neurotic disorders and physical complaints

There was a clear relationship between the number of neurotic disorders and the presence of any physical complaint; adults with one neurotic disorder were about one and a half times more likely to suffer a complaint than those with no disorder, and those with two or more disorders were almost twice as likely to have a physical complaint. This relationship was evident for men and women, but not for each type of physical complaint. *(Table 2.3, Figure 2.3)*

2.4 The type of neurotic disorder and physical complaints

Half of all adults with a disorder reported at least one physical complaint, and this proportion did not vary widely with the type of neurotic disorder; the proportions suffering any physical complaint ranged from 47% among those with Generalised Anxiety

Disorder or phobia, to 55% of those with Obsessive–Compulsive Disorder.

Although there were apparently large differences between adults with different neurotic disorders in the proportions suffering from particular physical complaints, these differences were not statistically significant. *(Table 2.4)*

2.5 Odds ratios of neurotic disorder associated with physical complaints

In order to investigate how the odds of having each physical complaint were associated with having a neurotic disorder, multiple logistic regression modelling was carried out, controlling for key socio-demographic and socio-economic factors: sex, age, ethnicity, employment status, qualifications, social class, family unit type, tenure, type of accommodation, and locality. *(Figure 2.4)*

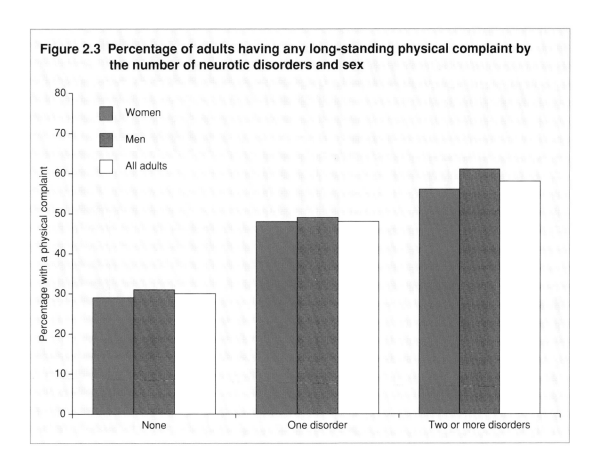

Figure 2.3 Percentage of adults having any long-standing physical complaint by the number of neurotic disorders and sex

Apart from eye complaints, ear complaints, or infectious and parasitic diseases, the presence of a neurotic disorder had a significant and positive association with the odds of each physical complaint. This is apparent as the 95% confidence intervals around the odds ratios encompass only values greater than one. (One is the baseline likelihood of having each physical complaint, given that no neurotic disorder is present.) Table 2.5 lists the other factors which, in addition to neurotic disorder, had a significant association with the odds of having each physical complaint.

Neurotic disorder had the greatest association with the odds of having genito-urinary complaints; odds were about five times higher among neurotic adults than their counterparts with no disorder (odds ratio = 4.77). Having a neurotic disorder more than doubled the odds of having digestive complaints (OR = 2.49), neoplasms (OR = 2.38) and musculo-skeletal complaints (OR = 2.31) compared with having

no neurotic disorder. *(Table 2.5, Figure 2.4)*

2.6 Neurotic disorders among adults with physical complaints

The discussion so far has concentrated on adults with neurotic disorders and looked at physical complaints in relation to having a neurotic disorder. The focus now turns to those adults who had a physical complaint and this section examines whether people with physical complaints were more likely than others to suffer a neurotic disorder.

Twice as many women and men with physical complaints had a neurotic disorder in contrast with their counterparts who had no physical complaints; 29% of women with a physical complaint had neurosis compared with 15% of women with neurosis and no physical complaint; for men the corresponding proportions were 19% and 9%.

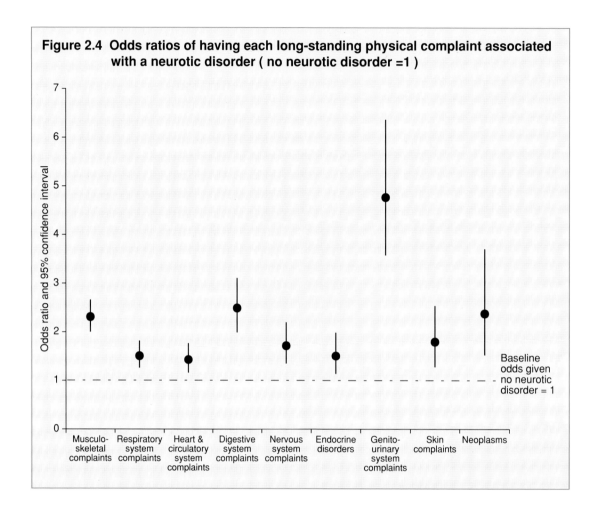

Figure 2.4 Odds ratios of having each long-standing physical complaint associated with a neurotic disorder (no neurotic disorder =1)

Compared with adults with other physical complaints, those with genito-urinary complaints had the greatest likelihood of having a neurotic disorder (47%), and this reflected the high proportion with neurosis among women who had this complaint (52%). There was also a greater likelihood of having a neurotic disorder among adults with neoplasms and digestive complaints than among those with other complaints (37% and 32% respectively).

Among adults with eye complaints, ear complaints or infectious and parasitic complaints, the proportions with a neurotic disorder were no different from those among adults with no physical complaint.

There were no differences according to the type of physical complaint in the proportions having one disorder or two or more disorders. *(Table 2.6, Figure 2.5)*

2.7 Physical complaints and worry about physical health

As part of the CIS–R, all adults were asked about the extent to which they worried about their physical health or about having a serious physical illness in the previous seven days. One point was assigned for each of the following criteria:

- The respondent worried for 4 or more days
- In the respondent's own opinion, he/she worried too much in view of his/her actual health
- The worrying had been very unpleasant
- The respondent had been unable to take his/her mind off these worries even once, by doing something else

A respondent with a score of two or more on this section of the CIS–R was defined as having

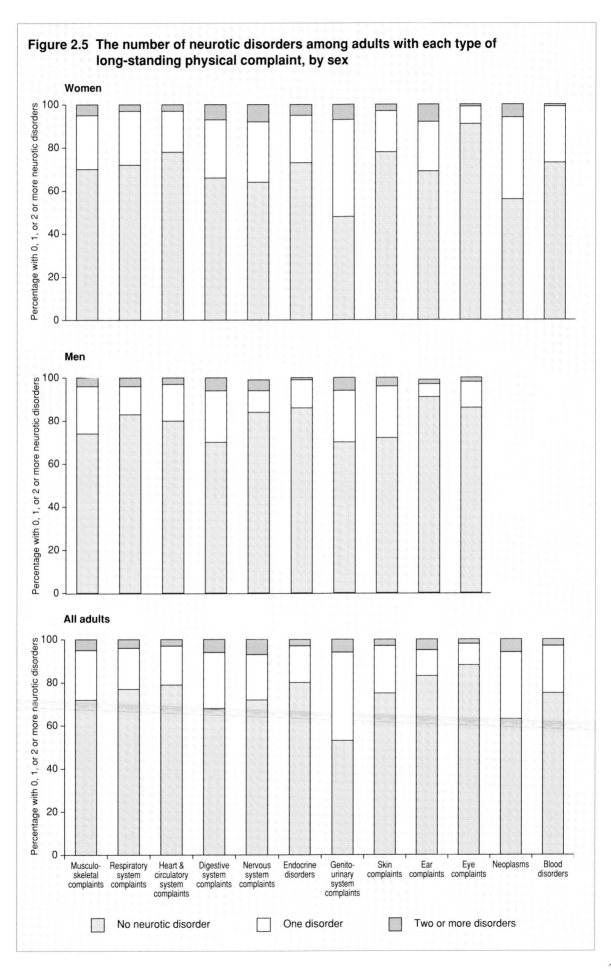

Figure 2.5 The number of neurotic disorders among adults with each type of long-standing physical complaint, by sex

significant symptoms of worry about physical health.

Table 2.7 shows the cumulative distribution of CIS–R scores on this symptom and how it varies by the type of physical condition. Overall, 4% of adults reported significant worry about their physical health, but 8% of those with a physical complaint reported such worry compared with 3% of those with no physical complaint.

Those with genito-urinary complaints were the most likely to worry about their physical health (16%) followed by those with neo-plasms, musculo-skeletal complaints or digestive complaints (11%). *(Table 2.7)*

References

1   Breeze, E., Trevor, G., Wilmot, A.,(1991) *General Household Survey Report 1989*, HMSO, London: Table 4.21.

2   *International Statistical Classification of Disorders and Related Health Problems 10th Revision* **Volume 1** (1992) WHO, Geneva.

Table 2.1 Percentage of adults with each physical complaint by neurotic disorder, compared with 1989 GHS estimates

	Any neurotic disorder	No neurotic disorder	All adults	GHS: adults aged 16-64
	Percentage with each complaint			
Musculo-skeletal complaints	23	11	13	11
Arthritis/rheumatism/fibrositis	9	4	5	
Back & neck problems/slipped disc	10	4	5	
Other problems of bones/joints/muscles	7	3	3	
Respiratory system complaints	10	7	7	6
Bronchitis/emphysema	1	1	1	
Asthma	7	4	4	
Hayfever	1	2	2	
Other respiratory complaints	2	1	1	
Heart and circulatory system complaints	8	5	6	5
Stroke and heart complaints	4	2	3	
Blood pressure complaints	3	3	3	
Blood vessel complaints	2	1	1	
Digestive system complaints	7	3	4	3
Stomach complaints & ulcers	4	1	2	
Large & small intestine complaints	3	1	2	
Other digestive complaints	0	1	0	
Nervous system complaints	6	3	3	3
Migraine	3	1	2	
Other nervous system complaints	3	2	2	
Endocrine disorders	4	3	3	2
Diabetes	2	1	1	
Hormone deficiency/thyroid disease /Addison's disease	2	1	1	
Other endocrine disorders	0	0	0	
Genito-urinary system complaints	6	1	2	2
Urinary tract/bladder/kidney complaints	2	1	1	
Reproductive system disorders	4	1	1	
Skin complaints	3	2	2	2
Ear complaints	2	2	2	2
Deafness	1	1	1	
Other ear complaints	1	1	1	
Eye complaints	1	1	1	1
Neoplasms	2	1	1	1
Blood disorders	1	0	1	0
Infectious and parasitic diseases	0	0	0	0
Any physical complaint	50	30	33	**
Base	*1557*	*8184*	*9741*	*15734*

** Information not available
Some adults had more than one complaint

Table 2.2 Long-standing physical complaints by age (grouped) by whether had a neurotic disorder and sex

Physical complaint	16-24	25-34	35-44	45-54	55-64	All
Women	*Percentage with each complaint*					
Any neurotic disorder						
Musculo-skeletal complaints	10	14	19	30	34	20
Respiratory system complaints	15	11	7	9	11	11
Heart & circulatory system complaints	1	3	7	10	11	6
Digestive system complaints	4	6	6	7	8	6
Nervous system complaints	5	8	8	7	8	7
Endocrine disorders	0	2	4	4	10	4
Genito-urinary system complaints	4	9	8	12	7	8
Skin complaints	2	3	1	1	2	2
Ear complaints	1	1	1	3	5	2
Eye complaints	-	0	0	0	2	0
Neoplasms	1	2	2	3	6	2
Blood disorders	1	1	0	1	1	1
Infectious & parasitic diseases	-	-	1	-	1	0
Any physical complaint	**35**	**44**	**49**	**61**	**63**	**49**
Base	*185*	*242*	*219*	*197*	*116*	*960*
No neurotic disorder						
Musculo-skeletal complaints	4	5	12	15	24	11
Respiratory system complaints	9	5	7	5	6	6
Heart & circulatory system complaints	1	1	4	7	16	5
Digestive system complaints	2	2	2	4	6	3
Nervous system complaints	2	2	5	3	4	3
Endocrine disorders	0	1	2	3	7	2
Genito-urinary system complaints	1	2	2	2	2	2
Skin complaints	3	2	1	1	1	2
Ear complaints	1	1	1	1	2	1
Eye complaints	1	0	1	1	1	1
Neoplasms	0	0	1	1	2	1
Blood disorders	1	0	1	1	0	1
Infectious & parasitic diseases	1	0	0	-	0	0
Any physical complaint	**20**	**18**	**30**	**32**	**49**	**29**
Base	*733*	*979*	*838*	*732*	*668*	*3948*
All women						
Musculo-skeletal complaints	5	7	13	18	25	13
Respiratory system complaints	10	6	7	6	7	7
Heart & circulatory system complaints	1	1	4	8	16	5
Digestive system complaints	2	2	3	4	6	4
Nervous system complaints	2	3	6	4	4	4
Endocrine disorders	0	1	2	3	7	3
Genito-urinary system complaints	2	4	3	4	2	3
Skin complaints	3	2	1	1	2	2
Ear complaints	1	1	1	1	2	1
Eye complaints	1	0	1	1	1	1
Neoplasms	0	1	1	1	2	1
Blood disorders	1	1	1	1	0	1
Infectious & parasitic diseases	0	0	0	0	0	0
Any physical complaint	**23**	**23**	**34**	**38**	**51**	**33**
Base	*917*	*1221*	*1057*	*929*	*784*	*4908*

Table 2.2 Long-standing physical complaints by age (grouped) by whether had a neurotic disorder and sex - *continued*

Physical complaint	16-24	25-34	35-44	45-54	55-64	All
Men	*percentage with each complaint*					
Any neurotic disorder						
Musculo-skeletal complaints	6	18	30	37	48	27
Respiratory system complaints	14	12	8	10	4	10
Heart & circulatory system complaints	-	2	7	15	33	10
Digestive system complaints	1	4	10	11	16	8
Nervous system complaints	2	3	3	7	2	3
Endocrine disorders	-	1	1	3	12	3
Genito-urinary system complaints	-	2	4	3	1	2
Skin complaints	2	8	5	2	1	4
Ear complaints	1	2	1	1	3	1
Eye complaints	1	2	2	1	2	2
Neoplasms	-	0	1	2	3	1
Blood disorders	2	-	-	-	1	1
Infectious & parasitic diseases	-	2	0	0	0	1
Any physical complaint	**23**	**41**	**53**	**64**	**73**	**50**
Base	*96*	*156*	*136*	*115*	*96*	*597*
No neurotic disorder						
Musculo-skeletal complaints	5	7	12	14	22	11
Respiratory system complaints	8	7	7	4	8	7
Heart & circulatory system complaints	1	1	2	9	20	6
Digestive system complaints	0	2	2	3	7	3
Nervous system complaints	2	3	3	3	3	3
Endocrine disorders	1	2	3	4	6	3
Genito-urinary system complaints	0	0	1	0	2	1
Skin complaints	2	2	2	1	1	2
Ear complaints	1	1	2	3	4	2
Eye complaints	2	1	1	2	2	1
Neoplasms	1	0	0	1	1	1
Blood disorders	-	0	0	-	1	0
Infectious & parasitic diseases	-	0	1	0	0	0
Any physical complaint	**19**	**23**	**29**	**35**	**55**	**31**
Base	*851*	*1063*	*864*	*800*	*658*	*4236*
All men						
Musculo-skeletal complaints	5	8	14	17	25	13
Respiratory system complaints	8	8	7	5	8	7
Heart & circulatory system complaints	1	1	3	10	22	6
Digestive system complaints	0	2	4	4	8	3
Nervous system complaints	2	3	3	3	3	3
Endocrine disorders	1	2	2	4	6	3
Genito-urinary system complaints	0	0	1	1	2	1
Skin complaints	2	2	2	1	2	2
Ear complaints	1	1	1	2	4	2
Eye complaints	2	1	1	2	2	1
Neoplasms	1	0	0	1	1	1
Blood disorders	0	0	0	0	1	0
Infectious & parasitic diseases	0	0	0	0	0	0
Any physical complaint	**20**	**25**	**32**	**38**	**57**	**33**
Base	*947*	*1219*	*1000*	*915*	*753*	*4833*

31

Table 2.2 Long-standing physical complaints by age (grouped) by whether had a neurotic disorder and sex - *continued*

Physical complaint	16-24	25-34	35-44	45-54	55-64	All
All adults	*Percentage with each complaint*					
Any neurotic disorder						
Musculo-skeletal complaints	8	15	23	33	40	23
Respiratory system complaints	15	11	8	10	8	10
Heart & circulatory system complaints	0	3	7	12	21	8
Digestive system complaints	3	5	8	9	12	7
Nervous system complaints	4	6	6	7	6	6
Endocrine disorders	0	2	3	4	11	4
Genito-urinary system complaints	2	6	6	8	4	6
Skin complaints	2	5	3	1	2	3
Ear complaints	1	1	1	2	4	2
Eye complaints	0	1	1	1	2	1
Neoplasms	1	1	2	2	4	2
Blood disorders	1	1	0	1	1	1
Infectious & parasitic diseases	0	1	0	0	1	0
Any physical complaint	**31**	**43**	**50**	**62**	**68**	**50**
Base	*280*	*398*	*355*	*312*	*212*	*1557*
No neurotic disorder						
Musculo-skeletal complaints	5	6	12	14	23	11
Respiratory system complaints	8	6	7	5	7	7
Heart & circulatory system complaints	1	1	3	8	18	5
Digestive system complaints	1	2	2	3	6	3
Nervous system complaints	2	2	4	3	3	3
Endocrine disorders	1	1	2	3	6	3
Genito-urinary system complaints	1	1	1	1	2	1
Skin complaints	2	2	2	1	1	2
Ear complaints	1	1	1	2	3	2
Eye complaints	1	1	1	1	2	1
Neoplasms	0	0	1	1	1	1
Blood disorders	0	0	0	0	1	0
Infectious & parasitic diseases	0	0	0	0	0	0
Any physical complaint	**19**	**20**	**30**	**34**	**52**	**30**
Base	*1584*	*2041*	*1702*	*1532*	*1325*	*8184*
All adults						
Musculo-skeletal complaints	5	8	14	18	25	13
Respiratory system complaints	9	7	7	6	7	7
Heart & circulatory system complaints	1	1	4	8	19	6
Digestive system complaints	1	2	3	4	7	4
Nervous system complaints	2	3	4	4	4	3
Endocrine disorders	1	2	2	3	7	3
Genito-urinary system complaints	1	2	2	2	2	2
Skin complaints	2	2	2	1	1	2
Ear complaints	1	1	1	2	3	2
Eye complaints	1	1	1	1	2	1
Neoplasms	0	0	1	1	2	1
Blood disorders	0	0	0	0	1	0
Infectious & parasitic diseases	0	0	0	0	0	0
Any physical complaint	**21**	**24**	**33**	**38**	**54**	**33**
Base	*1864*	*2439*	*2056*	*1844*	*1537*	*9741*

Some adults had more than one complaint.

Table 2.3 Longstanding physical complaints by number of neurotic disorders and sex

Physical complaint	Women			Men			All adults		
	None	One	Two or more	None	One or more	Two	None	One	Two or more
	Percentage with each complaint								
Musculo-skeletal complaints	11	19	28	11	27	28	11	22	28
Respiratory system complaints	6	11	9	7	9	18	7	10	12
Heart & circulatory system complaints	5	6	6	6	10	15	5	7	10
Digestive system complaints	3	6	9	3	8	12	3	6	10
Nervous system complaints	3	6	11	3	3	9	3	5	10
Endocrine disorders	2	3	5	3	3	1	3	3	4
Genito-urinary system complaints	2	8	8	1	2	3	1	6	6
Skin complaints	2	2	2	2	4	5	2	3	3
Ear complaints	1	2	3	2	1	3	2	1	3
Eye complaints	1	0	0	1	2	2	1	1	1
Neoplasms	1	2	3	1	1	2	1	2	2
Blood disorders	1	1	0	0	0	1	0	1	1
Infectious & parasitic diseases	0	0	0	0	0	1	0	0	1
Any physical complaint	**29**	**48**	**56**	**31**	**49**	**61**	**30**	**48**	**58**
Base	*3948*	*830*	*130*	*4236*	*519*	*79*	*8184*	*1348*	*209*

Some adults had more than one complaint.

Table 2.4 Longstanding physical complaints by neurotic disorder and sex

	Mixed anxiety and depressive disorder	Generalised Anxiety Disorder	Depressive episode	All phobias	Obsessive-Compulsive Disorder	Panic disorder	Any neurotic disorder	No neurotic disorder	All
	Percentage with each complaint								
Women									
Musculo-skeletal complaints	20	21	25	18	28	21	20	11	13
Respiratory system complaints	11	9	6	17	11	10	11	6	7
Heart & circulatory system complaints	6	7	5	8	5	7	6	5	5
Digestive system complaints	6	8	6	8	7	9	6	3	4
Nervous system complaints	7	8	7	11	10	5	7	3	4
Endocrine disorders	3	4	5	5	3	8	4	2	3
Genito-urinary system complaints	9	10	8	4	6	8	8	2	3
Skin complaints	2	1	2	4	2	4	2	2	2
Ear complaints	1	3	2	1	2	4	2	1	1
Eye complaints	0	0	1	0	-	1	0	1	1
Neoplasms	2	2	2	2	4	8	2	1	1
Blood disorders	1	1	0	0	1	-	1	1	1
Infectious & parasitic diseases	0	0	0	1	-	-	0	0	0
Any physical complaint	**52**	**48**	**47**	**49**	**57**	**50**	**49**	**29**	**33**
Base	*485*	*251*	*133*	*122*	*100*	*50*	*960*	*3948*	*4908*
Men									
Musculo-skeletal complaints	32	22	29	16	33	27	27	11	13
Respiratory system complaints	11	10	11	13	11	13	10	7	7
Heart & circulatory system complaints	10	14	14	8	7	6	10	6	7
Digestive system complaints	6	10	12	10	10	10	8	3	34
Nervous system complaints	3	3	10	8	4	-	3	3	3
Endocrine disorders	4	2	5	3	1	-	3	3	3
Genito-urinary system complaints	1	2	5	1	1	3	2	1	1
Skin complaints	5	3	6	6	6	-	4	2	2
Ear complaints	1	2	2	1	2	1	1	2	2
Eye complaints	2	1	1	5	3	1	2	1	1
Neoplasms	1	-	-	2	2	4	1	1	1
Blood disorders	1	-	1	2	-	-	1	0	0
Infectious & parasitic diseases	1	-	1	-	-	2	1	0	0
Any physical complaint	**56**	**45**	**60**	**44**	**50**	**51**	**50**	**31**	**33**
Base	*265*	*188*	*88*	*58*	*57*	*43*	*597*	*4236*	*4833*
All adults									
Musculo-skeletal complaints	24	22	26	18	30	24	23	11	13
Respiratory system complaints	11	9	8	16	11	11	10	7	7
Heart & circulatory system complaints	7	10	9	8	5	7	8	5	6
Digestive system complaints	6	9	8	9	8	9	7	3	4
Nervous system complaints	5	6	8	10	8	3	6	3	3
Endocrine disorders	4	3	5	4	2	5	4	3	3
Genito-urinary system complaints	6	7	7	3	4	6	6	1	2
Skin complaints	3	2	4	4	3	2	3	2	2
Ear complaints	1	3	2	1	2	2	2	2	2
Eye complaints	1	1	1	2	1	1	1	1	1
Neoplasms	2	1	2	2	3	6	2	1	1
Blood disorders	1	0	1	1	0	-	1	0	0
Infectious & parasitic diseases	0	0	1	1	-	1	0	0	0
Any physical complaint	**53**	**47**	**52**	**47**	**55**	**50**	**50**	**30**	**33**
Base	*750*	*439*	*220*	*180*	*157*	*93*	*1557*	*8184*	*9741*

Some adults had more than one complaint.

Table 2.5   Odds ratios of each long-standing physical complaint associated with having a neurotic disorder

Physical complaint	Adjusted Odds Ratio associated with neurotic disorder (cf no neurotic disorder)	95% CI	Other factors entered in model giving ORs which were:	
			Significant	Non–significant
Musculo–skeletal complaints	2.31***	(2.00–2.66)	Age, sex, family unit type, employment status, social class	Ethnicity, qualifications tenure, type of accommodation, locality
Respiratory system complaints	1.51***	(1.26–1.82)	Family unit type, employment status	Age, sex, ethnicity, qualifications, tenure, type of accommodation, social class, locality
Heart & circulatory system complaints	1.43**	(1.16–1.77)	Age, sex, qualifications, employment status, type of accommodation	Ethnicity, family unit type, tenure, social class, locality
Digestive system complaints	2.49***	(1.99–3.11)	Age	Sex, ethnicity, family unit type, qualifications, employment status, tenure, type of accommodation, social class, locality
Nervous system complaints	1.72***	(1.35–2.20)	Age, employment status, qualifications, type of accommodation	Sex, ethnicity, family unit type, tenure, social class locality
Endocrine disorders	1.51**	(1.14–1.99)	Age, ethnicity, employment status, social class	Sex, family unit type, qualifications, tenure, type of accommodation, locality
Genito–urinary system complaints	4.77***	(3.58–6.37)	Sex, age	Ethnicity, family unit type, qualifications, employment status, tenure, type of accommodation, social class, locality
Skin complaints	1.80***	(1.28–2.54)	—	All others
Neoplasms	2.38***	(1.53–3.71)	Sex, age, employment status	Ethnicity, family unit type, qualifications, social class, tenure, type of accommodation, locality

* p<0.05   ** p<0.01   ***p<0.001

The presence of a neurotic disorder did not have a significant association with the odds of having eye complaints, ear complaints, or infectious and parasitic diseases.

Table 2.6 Number of neurotic disorders by long-standing physical complaint and sex

	Musculo-skeletal complaints	Respiratory system complaints	Heart and circulatory system complaints	Digestive system complaints	Nervous system complaints	Endocrine disorders	Genito-urinary system complaints	Skin complaints
Women	%	%	%	%	%	%	%	%
No neurotic disorder	70	72	78	66	64	73	48	78
One disorder	25	25	19	27	28	22	45	19
Two or more disorders	6	3	3	7	8	5	7	3
Base	*638*	*358*	*260*	*174*	*188*	*132*	*150*	*88*
Men	%	%	%	%	%	%	%	%
No neurotic disorder	74	83	80	70	84	86	70	72
One disorder	22	13	17	24	10	13	24	24
Two or more disorders	4	4	4	6	5	1	6	4
Base	*632*	*349*	*303*	*165*	*128*	*132*	*39*	*90*
All adults	%	%	%	%	%	%	%	%
No neurotic disorder	72	77	79	68	72	80	53	75
One disorder	23	19	18	26	21	17	41	22
Two or more disorders	5	4	4	6	7	3	7	4
Base	*1269*	*706*	*563*	*339*	*316*	*263*	*190*	*177*

	Ear complaints	Eye complaints	Neoplasms	Blood disorders	Infectious & parasitic diseases	Any physical illness	No physical illness	All adults
Women	%	%	%	%	%	%	%	%
No neurotic disorder	69	91	56	73	[7]	71	85	80
One disorder	23	8	38	26	[2]	25	13	17
Two or more disorders	8	1	7	2	[0]	5	2	3
Base	*53*	*37*	*52*	*30*	*10*	*1610*	*3298*	*4908*
Men	%	%	%	%	%	%	%	%
No neurotic disorder	91	86	[20]	[12]	[9]	81	91	88
One disorder	6	12	[5]	[2]	[2]	16	8	11
Two or more disorders	2	2	[1]	[1]	[1]	3	1	2
Base	*93*	*68*	*27*	*15*	*12*	*1595*	*3238*	*4833*
All adults	%	%	%	%	%	%	%	%
No neurotic disorder	83	88	63	75	[17]	76	88	84
One disorder	12	10	31	22	[4]	20	11	14
Two or more disorders	5	2	6	3	[2]	4	1	2
Base	*146*	*105*	*79*	*45*	*22*	*3206*	*6535*	*9741*

Table 2.7   Cumulative CIS-R scores for worry about physical health by long-standing physical complaint

Cumulative CIS-R score for worry about physical health	Musculo-skeletal complaints	Respiratory system complaints	Heart and circulatory system complaints	Digestive system complaints	Nervous system complaints	Endocrine disorders	Genito-urinary system complaints	Skin complaints
Cumulative percentage								
4	1	0	0	1	0	0	1	1
3 or more	3	2	2	3	3	2	6	3
2 or more	11	5	9	11	8	9	16	7
1 or more	23	16	19	23	18	20	32	21
0 or more	100	100	100	100	100	100	100	100
Base	*1269*	*706*	*563*	*339*	*316*	*263*	*190*	*177*

Cumulative CIS-R score for worry about physical health	Ear complaints	Eye complaints	Neoplasms	Blood disorders diseases	Infectious & parasitic illness	Any physical illness	No physical	All adults
4	0	0	0	0	[0]	0	0	0
3 or more	1	0	6	2	[0]	2	1	1
2 or more	6	5	11	2	[2]	8	3	4
1 or more	14	13	29	10	[7]	18	8	12
0 or more	100	100	100	100	[22]	100	100	100
Base	*146*	*105*	*79*	*45*	*22*	*3206*	*6535*	*9741*

3 Medication and other forms of treatment

3.1 Introduction

This chapter looks at the extent to which people identified as having a neurotic illness were on medication or other forms of treatment. At the most general level, two types of psychotropic medication are described: antidepressants, and hypnotics and anxiolytics. At the most specific level, particular classes of drugs were identified (based on the British National Formulary).[1]

Antidepressants

- Tricyclic antidepressants
- Monoamine oxidase inhibitors
- Compound antidepressants
- Other antidepressants, mainly serotonin reuptake inhibitors

Hypnotics and anxiolytics

- Hypnotics
- Anxiolytics

Other forms of treatment are also subsumed under two broad categories, therapy and counselling. Although the interview sought to identify the precise type of treatment, most responses were of a general nature. Therefore, the two categories therapy and counselling are predominantly used in the analysis.

Therapy

- Psychotherapy, psychoanalysis, individual or group therapy, analysis, talking with psychiatrist, visit by therapist
- Behaviour or cognitive therapy
- Sex, marital or family therapy
- Art, music or drama therapy
- Social skills training

Counselling

- Counselling, talking to social worker or community psychiatric nurse or Samaritans, rape crisis centre, Alcoholics Anonymous, talking to doctor or psychologist for counselling.

3.2 Use of medication or treatment

About 1 in 8 people with a neurotic disorder were having treatment. Among this group, two thirds were taking medication and a half were having either therapy or counselling. A small proportion of people had both sorts of treatment.

Those classified as having two or more neurotic disorders were three times more likely to have received some form of treatment than those with one disorder (30% compared with 10%). If number of disorders is regarded as a measure of the overall severity of neurosis, then those with a more severe disorder were four times as likely to be on medication and twice as likely to be receiving counselling or therapy. *(Table 3.1)*

It is interesting to note that among the sample of 8184 adults without a neurotic disorder, only 7 were taking antidepressants and 13, anxiolytics or hypnotics. At one level, this indicates the success of the CIS–R in identifying neurotic psychopathology. At another, it suggests that there is little overprescription of treatment of those without significant neurotic symptoms: good practice advises that patients remain on antidepressants for up to 6 months after full recovery from depression to prevent relapse.

Questions on counselling and therapy were only asked of those who had a neurotic disorder.

Table 3.2 shows that the groups most likely to be receiving treatment were those classified as having a phobia (28%) or a depressive episode (25%); those least likely to be having treatment were those with mixed anxiety and depressive disorder (9%). This may be due to the greater degree of psychiatric comorbidity between depression or phobia with other neurotic disorders, as shown in Chapter 1, and to the relative mildness of the residual condition. *(Table 3.2)*

Tables 3.3 and 3.4 show the distribution of use of particular classes of medication or types of therapy or counselling among those receiving treatment. For those on antidepressants, the majority were taking tricyclic antidepressants, the remainder were taking a class of drug categorised by the BNF as 'other depressants' of which the majority were serotonin uptake inhibitors. Among those taking hypnotics and anxiolytics, about a half were taking each type of medication. Clearly, some people are taking both types. *(Table 3.3)*

Treatment by therapy or counselling was also equally distributed among those having such treatment. *(Table 3.4)*

3.3 Odds ratios of factors associated with having treatment

Multiple logistic regression was used as a method of identifying the factors which increased the odds of having treatment compared with those who did not, among respondents who had neurotic disorders. The analysis was carried out for six dependent variables:

(i)   taking antidepressants
(ii) taking hypnotics or anxiolytics
(iii) taking any antidepressant, hypnotic or anxiolytic
(iv) having therapy
(v)   having counselling
(vi) having therapy or counselling

Factors entered in the analysis were those socio-demographic characteristics which were found to increase the odds of having a neurotic disorder: sex, age, ethnicity, family unit type, employment status, tenure and locality.[2] Other factors entered in the model were the number of neurotic disorders, whether the person also had a longstanding limiting physical illness, number of stressful life events and a measure of perceived social support.

The number of neurotic disorders was included because those with more than one disorder were more likely to have medication or other forms of treatment. The experience of at least one stressful life event seemed an appropriate choice as it was hypothesised that those who had suffered such an event in the past six months may have sought treatment to cope with the impact of the stressful event. Perceived social support was included because it was felt that those with no-one to turn to may seek medication or therapy whereas those with a good social support network may turn to their family and friends for help instead of seeking professional help.

Tables 3.5 to 3.10 show that the main factor which increased the odds of getting any medication was having more than one neurotic disorder. The effect of having two or more neurotic disorders was most pronounced for taking antidepressants (OR = 4.85, p<0.001). Comorbid neurotic disorders also increased the odds of having counselling (OR = 2.95, p<0.001). *(Tables 3.5 to 3.10)*

Among the socio-demographic variables which emerged as increasing the odds of having particular treatments, age had the most striking effect. Compared with the reference group of 16–24 year olds those in older age groups had progressively higher odds of taking anxiolytics and hypnotics. For the oldest age group the odds ratio was 8.93 (p<0.01). *(Table 3.6)*

3.4 Compliance with medicinal regimes

Two in five of those adults on antidepressants,

hypnotics or anxiolytics said that they sometimes did not take their medication when they knew they should; just over half of them had not taken their medicine in the past week. Forgetfulness, feeling the medication was not needed, dislike of taking drugs, and side-effects were all mentioned as reasons for non-compliance.

3.5 Previous treatment

About half of the 133 adults with a neurotic disorder who were on antidepressants, hypnotics or anxiolytics, had tried other treatment. Among the group who had previous treatment, three quarters had stopped on professional advice, a quarter gave up treatment on their own accord.

3.6 Refusal of treatment

Only those who were presently having treatment, drugs, therapy or counselling, were asked whether they had been offered treatment which they refused. Only one in ten had refused treatment. Numbers are too small to comment on what was refused and the reasons for refusal.

3.7 Comorbid physical illness and its treatment

In Chapter 2 the extent of comorbidity between physical illness and neurotic disorders was demonstrated. This is also reflected in the medication taken for those physical illnesses. In Table 3.11 medicines taken by those who have both a neurotic disorder and a physical illness are grouped together according to the BNF chapter headings, which in many but not all cases relate to systems of bodily functioning (digestion, respiration, circulation, etc).

About a third of those who had a neurotic disorder and reported having a longstanding, physical illness were taking medication for nervous system problems (31%). Drugs for cardiovascular, gastro-intestinal, respiratory, endocrine and musculo-skeletal systems were also taken by 10 to 15 per cent of those with a neurotic disorder. This distribution is similar to that found among those with a physical illness and no neurotic disorder, with the exception of CNS drugs.

References

1. *British National Formulary* Number 26, September 1993, A joint publication of the British Medical Association and the Royal Pharmaceutical Society of Great Britain.

2. Meltzer, H., Gill, B., Petticrew, M., and Hinds, K. (1995) *OPCS surveys of Psychiatric Morbidity in Great Britian, Report 1, The prevalence of psychiatric morbidity among adults living in private households*, HMSO, London.

Table 3.1 Type of treatment by number of neurotic disorders

	Number of disorders		
	One neurotic disorder	Two or more neurotic disorders	Any neurotic disorder
	Percentage of adults with each type of treatment		
Any medication	**6**	**25**	**9**
Antidepressants	4	18	6
Anxiolytics and hypnotics	3	12	4
Any counselling or therapy	**5**	**12**	**6**
Counselling	2	7	3
Therapy	2	6	3
Any treatment	**10**	**30**	**12**
Base	*1348*	*209*	*1557*
Medication only	5	17	6
Counselling or therapy only	3	5	4
Both types of treatment	1	8	2

Table 3.2 Type of treatment by type of neurotic disorder

	Mixed anxiety and depressive disorder	Generalised Anxiety Disorder	Depressive episode	Phobia	Obsessive-Compulsive Disorder	Panic	Any neurotic disorder
	Percentage of adults with each type of treatment						
Any medication	**6**	**12**	**21**	**21**	**16**	**13**	**9**
Antidepressants	3	8	16	15	12	11	6
Anxiolytics and hypnotics	2	7	10	11	9	3	4
Any counselling or therapy	**4**	**7**	**11**	**14**	**9**	**6**	**6**
Counselling	2	3	6	8	5	3	3
Therapy	2	4	5	7	3	3	3
Any treatment	**9**	**16**	**25**	**28**	**19**	**15**	**12**
Base	*750*	*439*	*220*	*180*	*157*	*93*	*1557*
Medication only	5	9	14	14	11	9	6
Counselling or therapy only	3	3	4	7	3	2	4
Both types of treatment	1	3	7	7	5	4	2

Table 3.3 Type of medication by number of neurotic disorders

	Number of disorders		
	One neurotic disorder	Two or more disorders	Any neurotic disorder
	Percentage of adults taking each type of medication		
Any antidepressant	62	74	67
Tricyclic antidepressants	48	48	48
Monoamine oxidase inhibitors	1	1	1
Compound antidepressants	-	-	-
Other antidepressants, mainly serotonin reuptake inhibitors	13	25	18
Any anxiolytic or hypnotic	47	49	48
Anxiolytics	22	35	27
Hypnotics	26	20	24
Base (= people on medication)	*81*	*52*	*133*

Table 3.4 Type of therapy or counselling by number of neurotic disorders

	Number of disorders		
	One neurotic disorder	Two or more disorders	Any neurotic disorder
	Percentage of adults with each type of treatment		
Psychotherapy, psychoanalysis, individual or group therapy, etc	41	[9]	39
	-	-	-
Behaviour or cognitive therapy	2	-	2
Sex, marital or family therapy	3	-	2
Art, music or drama therapy	2	-	2
Social skills training	3	[3]	5
Counselling	48	[15]	51
Base (= people having therapy or counselling)	*65*	*25*	*91*

Table 3.5 Odds ratios associated with treatment by antidepressants

Factors	Adjusted ORs	95% CI
Number of neurotic disorders		
One	1.00	....
Two or more	4.85***	(3.04–7.73)
Age		
16-24	1.00	....
25-34	1.49	(0.60–3.71)
35-44	2.66**	(1.12–6.33)
45-54	3.19**	(1.37–7.47)
55-64	1.86	(0.73–4.74)
Employment status		
Working full time	1.00	....
Working part time	0.93	(0.42–2.07)
Unemployed	1.27	(0.58–2.78)
Economically inactive	2.35*	(1.32–4.13)
Physical illness		
No	1.00	....
Yes	1.62*	(1.00–2.64)

* p<0.05;   ** p<0.01;   *** p<0.001

Table 3.6 Odds ratios associated with treatment by anxiolytics or hypnotics

Factors	Adjusted ORs	95% CI
Number of neurotic disorders		
One	1.00	....
Two or more	4.04***	(2.32–7.04)
Age		
16–24	1.00	....
25–34	1.04	(0.20–5.44)
35–44	4.78*	(1.10–20.68)
45–54	7.50**	(1.76–32.00)
55–64	8.93**	(2.04–38.98)
Family type		
Couple no child(ren)	1.00	....
Couple and child(ren)	0.70	(0.32–1.54)
Lone parent and child(ren)	1.40	(0.51–3.82)
One person only	2.79	(1.40–5.59)
Adult with parents	2.32	(0.39–13.69)
Adult with one parent	0.86	(0.05–15.74)
Physical illness		
No	1.00	....
Yes	2.42**	(1.31–4.51)

* p<0.05;   ** p<0.01;   *** p<0.001

Table 3.7 Odds ratios associated with treatment by any medication

Factors	Adjusted ORs	95% CI
Number of neurotic disorders		
One	1.00	....
Two or more	4.54***	(3.02–6.82)
Age		
16–24	1.00	....
25–34	1.19	(0.53–2.66)
35–44	2.71**	(1.29–5.70)
45–54	3.67***	(1.78–7.57)
55–64	2.81**	(1.30–6.11)
Emploment status		
Working full time	1.00	....
Working part time	1.03	(0.55–1.92)
Unemployed	0.97	(0.49–1.92)
Economically inactive	1.95**	(1.21–3.13)
Physical illness		
No	1.00	....
Yes	1.81**	(1.20–2.74)

* p<0.05; ** p<0.01; *** p<0.001)

Table 3.8 Odds ratios associated with treatment by counselling

Factors	Adjusted ORs	95% CI
Number of neurotic disorders		
One	1.00	....
Two or more	2.95***	(1.55–5.61)
Employment status		
Working full time	1.00	....
Working part time	0.18	(0.03–1.11)
Unemployed	1.72	(0.77–3.86)
Economically inactive	1.4	(0.70–2.79)

* p<0.05; ** p<0.01; *** p<0.001)

Table 3.9 Odds ratios associated with treatment by therapy

Factors	Adjusted ORs	95% CI
Employment status		
Working full time	1.00	....
Working part time	0.27	(0.05–1.49)
Unemployed	3.06**	(1.38–6.78)
Economically inactive	2.14*	(1.04–4.40)

* p<0.05; ** p<0.01; *** p<0.001)

Table 3.10 Odds ratios associated with treatment by counselling or therapy

Factors	Adjusted ORs	95% CI
Number of neurotic disorders		
One	1.00	....
Two or more	2.35***	(1.43–3.86)
Employment status		
Working full time	1.00	....
Working part time	0.22*	(0.06–0.76)
Unemployed	1.97*	(1.08–3.57)
Economically inactive	1.56	(0,93–2.60)
Perceived social support		
No lack	1.00	....
Moderate lack	1.74*	(1.05–2.87)
Severe lack	1.97*	(1.13–3.41)

* p<0.05; ** p<0.01; *** p<0.001

Table 3.11 Type of medication taken by adults with neurotic disorders who also have physical illness

	Mixed anxiety and depressive disorder	Generalised Anxiety Disorder	Depressive episode	Phobia	Obsessive - Compulsive Disorder	Panic	Any neurotic disorder	No neurotic disorder
	%	%	%	%	%	%	%	%
Gastro-intestinal system drugs	8	12	11	13	12	10	10	7
Cardio-vascular system drugs	11	17	13	13	7	18	13	16
Respiratory system drugs	13	13	13	28	11	18	14	13
Central nervous system drugs*	28	38	46	47	38	30	31	14
Anti-infection drugs	4	2	4	9	4	4	4	3
Endocrine system drugs	9	16	10	12	12	17	11	9
Genito-urinary system drugs	1	1	-	3	-	3	1	2
Malignant drugs or immunosuppressants	0	1	1	-	1	-	0	0
Drugs used for nutrition and blood	2	4	3	3	2	6	3	2
Musculo-skeletal system drugs	14	17	20	18	20	16	15	10
Base	*399*	*207*	*115*	*85*	*86*	*47*	*773*	*2433*

* Apart from anxiolytics, hypnotics and antidepressants, the other main CNS drugs used were analgesics.

4 Use of services

4.1 Introduction

This chapter examines the use of health and other services by adults aged 16 to 64 years with a neurotic disorder. The use of some services is examined in relation to the presence of neurotic disorder, and to the sex of the informant. GP consultations and in-patient stays are also presented by type of neurotic disorder.

The types of services used by people with neurotic disorders are grouped into four categories: GP consultations (section 4.2), in-patient episodes (section 4.3), out-patient visits (section 4.4) and visits to peoples homes, for example, by a social or voluntary worker (section 4.5). A final section deals with services which people had been offered, but turned down (section 4.6).

4.2 GP consultations

GP consultations in past two weeks

All informants in the survey were asked about consultations for any reason in the past two weeks, and about consultations for physical complaints or for mental or emotional problems in the past year. Consultations either in person or by telephone were included but visits to a hospital were excluded. People with a neurotic disorder were in addition asked about consultations on their own behalf (as opposed to 'for any reason') in the past two weeks, and were asked about consultations for physical and mental health problems in the same period.

Overall, 20% of women and 13% of men in the sample had consulted a GP in the two weeks before interview, in line with the General Household Survey 1993 (GHS)[1] which found

20% of women and 12% of men aged 16 to 64 years had consulted within the same period. For both men and women with a neurotic disorder, the proportion consulting a GP for any reason in the past two weeks was twice that among those without a neurotic disorder. *(Table 4.1)*

Information on the reasons for consultations with GPs in the past two weeks was obtained from people with a neurotic disorder. In only a small percentage of this group had this consultation been for a mental health problem, or for a mental and physical complaint. However, almost one in four women and around one in seven men with neurotic disorders had consulted GPs for a physical complaint in the past two weeks. *(Table 4.2)*

People with neurotic disorders were asked whether they were satisfied or dissatisfied with their consultation. Twenty four per cent of these informants expressed dissatisfaction with their consultation for a mental problem. Dissatisfaction was lower (18%) when the consultation was for a physical health problem, and higher (31%) when the consultation involved both a physical and mental problem. The most common reason for dissatisfaction with either a physical or a mental consultation was that the doctor did not listen, the next most common being that the informant felt that the treatment was inappropriate.

The percentage of people with neurotic disorders consulting a GP in the past two weeks was also examined according to the type of disorder. This shows only minor differences between the disorders, though the percentage of people reporting a consultation was slightly higher among people with phobia or depressive episode. *(Figure 4.1)*

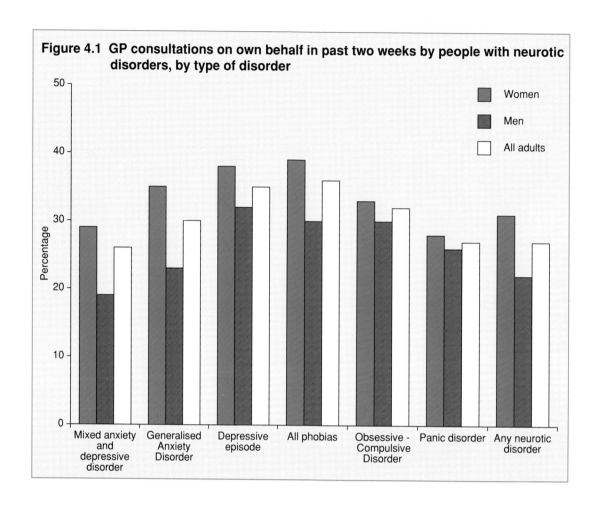

Figure 4.1 GP consultations on own behalf in past two weeks by people with neurotic disorders, by type of disorder

GP consultations in the past twelve months

All informants were also asked about GP consultations in the previous twelve months. Those with a neurotic disorder were more likely to have seen a GP for a physical complaint in this period. This finding is fairly consistent across all age groups and the pattern is also apparent in both sexes. For example, two thirds of women without a neurotic disorder, compared with over three quarters of women with a neurotic disorder, had seen a GP for a physical complaint during this period. Similarly, about half of men without a neurotic disorder and three quarters of those with a neurotic disorder had seen a GP for a physical problem during this reference period. This general association between GP consultations for a physical complaint and the presence of neurotic disorder is consistent with the higher prevalence of longstanding illness reported by

those with neurotic disorders than by those without, shown in Chapter 2.

Not surprisingly, the presence of neurotic disorder was strongly related to whether or not a GP had been consulted for a mental health problem in the past twelve months. Ten per cent of women with no neurotic disorder, compared with 40% of women with a disorder, had seen a GP; for men the relevant percentages were 5% and 27%. *(Table 4.1)*

Odds ratios of socio-demographic correlates of GP consultations

Multiple logistic regression was used to determine the relationship between GP consultations and a range of socio-demographic variables: sex, age, ethnic group, educational qualifications, family unit type, employment status, occupation type (manual, non-manual), type of accommodation, tenure and locality (urban, semi-rural/rural). Variables indicating the presence or absence of alcohol dependence, drug dependence, physical illness and neurotic disorder were also included in the model. Drug and alcohol dependence were assessed by means of a self-completion questionnaire, which can be found in Report 1 in this series.[2]

Three logistic regression models were produced to examine the effect of these variables on:

(i)   GP consultations for any reason in the past two weeks,

(ii) GP consultations for a physical complaint in the past twelve months, and

(iii) GP consultations for a mental complaint in the past twelve months.

Binary variables were created to indicate whether or not there had been a GP consultation. Odds ratios were then produced for each of the significant independent variables, to indicate the change in odds of a consultation associated with each of these variables, controlling for others in the model.

Odds ratios of GP consultations for any reason in the past two weeks

The odds of a GP consultation for any reason in the past two weeks were almost doubled by the presence of a neurotic disorder. The presence of physical illness increased the odds of a GP consultation by about half, while being female had a similar effect. The odds were increased by about one-third by being economically inactive, and were significantly decreased for adults living with parents. *(Table 4.3)*

Odds ratios of GP consultations for a physical health problem in the past year

Not surprisingly, the presence of a physical health problem had the largest effect of any variable on the odds of a GP consultation for a physical health problem (almost trebling them). The odds increased with age and the presence

of a neurotic disorder was associated with an increase in odds of a consultation about 40%.

The odds of a GP consultation for a physical health problem in the past twelve months were also increased by being female and being in the Asian or Oriental ethnic group. Economic inactivity and living in rented accommodation as opposed to being an owner-occupier both increased the odds of a consultation by around a quarter, while the odds were also increased by being in the group with no educational qualifications. Living in rented accommodation was associated with an increase in odds of 14%. *(Table 4.4)*

Odds ratios of GP consultations for a mental health problem

The presence of a neurotic disorder almost quadrupled the odds of a GP consultation for a mental problem, and the odds were more than doubled by being in the Asian or Oriental ethnic group. The presence of physical illness had a similar effect. An increase in odds was also associated with being female and with having any working status other than working full-time. Drug dependence increased the odds by almost two thirds, and being in any of the age groups between 25 and 54 was also associated with an increase in the odds of this type of consultation. *(Table 4.5)*

4.3 In-patient episodes during the past year

People with neurotic disorders were asked about in-patient stays in the past year. This referred to a stay in hospital of one night or longer for treatment or tests. In-patient stays for sight or hearing problems were included but hospitalisation while giving birth was excluded. Information on in-patient stays was not collected from people without neurotic disorders, so the GHS[1] has been used to provide comparable information for the adult population.

Fifteen per cent of women and 12% of men with

neurotic disorders had a hospital stay as an in-patient in the past year. This is higher than the percentages for the whole population found in the 1993 General Household Survey[1] , where 12% of women and 7% of men aged 16 to 64 years had been an in-patient in the previous twelve months. For some of the individual disorders the difference between the neurotic population and the general population in the same age group is even more marked, for example, 23% of people with a phobia and 21% of those with depressive episode had been an in-patient in the previous year. The percentage of women with panic disorder who had been in-patients in the past year is however slightly lower than in the general adult population. *(Figure 4.2)*

The majority of in-patient stays among people with neurotic disorders during the past year were for a physical health problem. A minority of people had more than one hospital stay during this period. *(Table 4.6, Table 4.7)*

The mean total length of stay (LOS) in the past year for people with neurotic disorders, 8 days, was the same as that found in the GHS.[1] The mean lengths of stay for women and men, 8 days and 10 days, were also similar to those found in the GHS, which found the mean LOS for women for any problem to be 7 days and the mean LOS for men to be 9 days. The mean LOS for mental health problems among people with neurotic disorders in this survey was 1 day.

The most common source of referral to hospital for mental health problems was a GP. GPs accounted for almost one third (31%) of these referrals, while about a fifth (19%) of patients were referred by a hospital casualty department. A similar proportion (19%) had admitted themselves. Psychiatrists or social workers had only been responsible for a small percentage of referrals.

Information on health professionals seen by the patient when in hospital was reported for 36

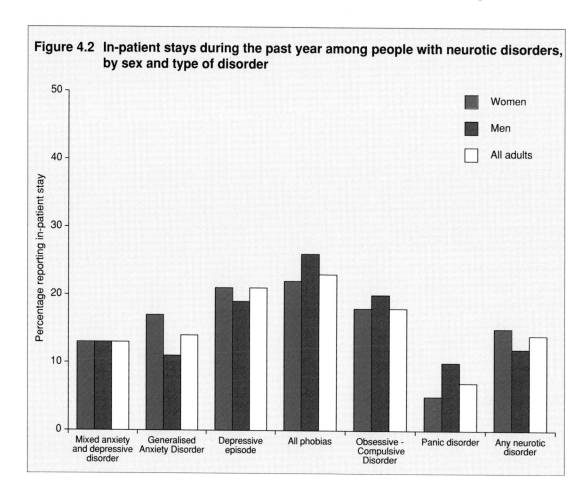

Figure 4.2   In-patient stays during the past year among people with neurotic disorders, by sex and type of disorder

hospital stays for a mental health problem. Excluding nurses with non-specific duties, the patient was most likely to recall having seen a psychiatrist or psychotherapist. In a third of these stays, patients recalled contact with one of these professionals, while a hospital doctor or consultant was apparently the next most frequent contact, patients having recalled contact during a quarter of hospital stays for a mental health problem. *(Table 4.8)*

4.4 Out-patient episodes in the past 12 months

For people with neurotic disorders, information was collected about visits to a hospital or clinic or anywhere else for treatment or check-ups. This included visits to hospitals, day hospitals, clinics and private consulting rooms. It also included attendance at day centres for treatment, but excluded attendance at day centres for leisure purposes, and sheltered workshops. Informants were also told to exclude visits to or from their own doctor, and to exclude periods when they stayed in
hospital.

Half of the men and women in this population had received treatment or check-ups in the past 12 months, and of those who had, the majority had been to just one place during that year for treatment. *(Table 4.9)*

The main reason for such visits was a physical health problem. Just less than half of informants had visited a hospital or clinic for this reason in the past year. By comparison, about one in twenty people cited a mental health problem as the reason for their visit.
(Table 4.10)

More than half of the people had their out-patient treatment or check-up at a hospital out-patient department. Other common places for such a visit were a clinic or health centre and private consulting rooms, which had been visited by about a fifth of those visiting for a

mental health problem. Only a small percentage of this group had attended a day centre or hospital casualty department. *(Table 4.11)*

About half of the patients visiting in connection with a mental health problem reported seeing a psychiatrist or psychotherapist. The next most frequently seen health professionals were psychologists, hospital doctors or consultants, and psychiatric nurses. *(Table 4.12)*

People who had stopped attending out-patients

The results discussed above apply to out-patient visits in the past twelve months. However most people who attended such a place over the past year were not currently doing so: only about 3% of people reported that they were currently attending, compared to 50% who reported an attendance at some time over the past year. Of those who had stopped attending in connection with a mental health problem, 60% had stopped of their own accord, as opposed to having been discharged.

4.5 Domiciliary visits in the past year

Informants were asked whether they had received a visit in their home from one of the following sources:

- Community Psychiatric Nurse (CPN)
- Occupational Therapist (OT)
- Social worker
- Psychiatrist
- Home care worker/home help
- Voluntary worker

Eight per cent of women and men with neurotic disorders had such a visit in the past year. Four per cent had a visit from a social worker, and 1% of people had a visit from each of the other types of helper. With the exception of home care workers, the helper usually came once a month or less often. Home care workers/home helps were more likely to visit on a weekly basis.

4.6 People who had refused help or support

Informants with a neurotic disorder were asked whether they had been offered any help or support in the past year which they had turned down. Only about 6% of this group had done so, with the most common source of help refused being a social worker. This may be simply because informants are most likely to be offered help from that source. *(Table 4.13)*

The most common reason for refusing help was that the informant did not want help, or felt that they did not need it; almost half the people with a neurotic disorder who had turned down help gave this as a reason. A quarter gave as a reason for refusal that they did not think the support they were offered

would be helpful, and about one in ten people refused because they could not face receiving help or support. Only a small minority of people refused help because it was inconvenient in terms of timing or location. *(Table 4.14)*

Informants were asked whether they had not seen a doctor or other professional about a mental, nervous or emotional problem, when either they or those around them thought they should. Twenty-five per cent of people with neurotic disorders reported that they had not sought help under these circumstances in the past year. The proportion deciding not to seek help was roughly the same for men and women (23% and 26% respectively).

The two most commonly stated reasons for not seeing a doctor or other professional were that the informant did not think anyone could help, and that they themselves should be able to cope with their problem. Fear of the consequences of seeking help, such as fear of side effects or of

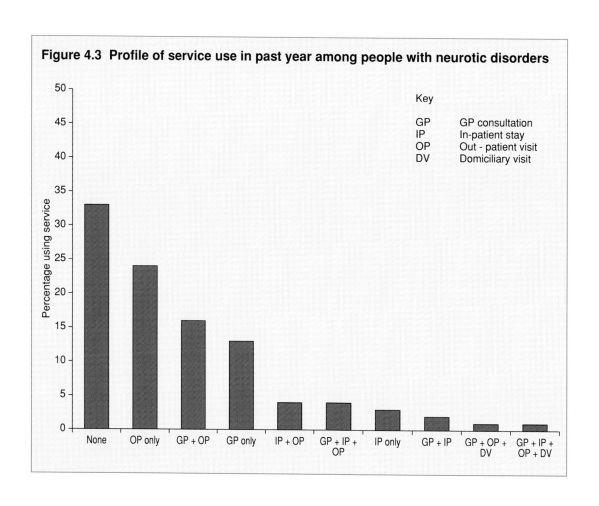

Figure 4.3 Profile of service use in past year among people with neurotic disorders

Key

GP	GP consultation
IP	In-patient stay
OP	Out - patient visit
DV	Domiciliary visit

treatment, tests or being sectioned, was much less common. Fear of friends' or family's reaction was given as a reason for not seeking help by 4%, but only 1% of informants actually did not seek help because of objections from their family or friends. Only 3% of informants had not sought help with a mental problem because they did not know who to go to, or where to go. *(Table 4.15)*

4.7 Profile of service use

An overall profile of service use among people with neurotic disorders (based on the four categories of services described above) shows that two thirds of this group had used some of these services in the past year. The majority (37%) had used a GP and at least one other service during this period. For people using two

services only, the most common combination was a GP consultation in the past two weeks, with an out-patient visit during the past year. Five per cent of people had used three different services in the past year, and only 1% had used a combination of all four services. *(Figure 4.3)*

References

1. Foster, K, Jackson, B., Thomas, M., Hunter, P., Bennett, N., (1995) *General Household Survey 1993*, HMSO, London.

2. Meltzer, H., Gill, B., Petticrew, M. & Hinds, K., (1995) *OPCS Surveys of Psychiatric Morbidity in Great Britain, Report 1, The prevalence of psychiatric morbidity among adults aged 16-64 living in private households in Great Britain.* HMSO, London.

Table 4.1 GP consultations by presence of neurotic disorder and sex

	Any neurotic disorder	No neurotic disorder	All
	Percentage consulting GPs		
Women			
Consulted GP in past two weeks for any reason	33	17	20
Consulted GP in past twelve months for physical complaint	80	66	68
Consulted GP in past twelve months for mental complaint	40	10	16
Base	*960*	*3948*	*4908*
Men			
Consulted GP in past two weeks for any reason	23	12	13
Consulted GP in past twelve months for physical complaint	74	58	60
Consulted GP in past twelve months for mental complaint	27	5	8
Base	*597*	*4236*	*4833*
All adults			
Consulted GP in past two weeks for any reason	29	14	16
Consulted GP in past twelve months for physical complaint	78	62	64
Consulted GP in past twelve months for mental complaint	35	7	12
Base	*1557*	*8184*	*9741*

Table 4.2   Reasons for consultations on own behalf by individuals with neurotic disorders during past two weeks

	Consultation for physical complaint	Consultation for mental problem	Consultation for both	*Base*
Women				
% consulting	23	3	4	*874*
Total % consulting		31		
Men				
% consulting	16	2	4	*521*
Total % consulting		22		
All				
% consulting	20	3	4	*1396*
Total % consulting		27		

The overall base of people with neurotic disorders (1396) is lower in this chapter than in previous chapters as 161 people who should have received a long interview covering service use did not.

Table 4.3   Odds ratios of socio–demographic correlates of GP consultations for any reason in past two weeks

	Adjusted OR	(95% CI)
Neurotic disorder		
Absent	1.00	....
Present	1.86**	(1.54–2.22)
Physical illness		
Absent	1.00	....
Present	1.54**	(1.25–1.89)
Sex		
Male	1.00	....
Female	1.52**	(1.35–1.73)
Employment status		
Working full time	1.00	....
Working part time	0.95	(0.80–1.13)
Unemployed	1.22	(1.00–1.50)
Economically inactive	1.32**	(1.15–1.53)
Family unit type		
Couple, no children	1.00	....
Couple & child(ren)	0.98	(0.85–1.12)
Lone parent & child(ren)	0.89	(0.70–1.14)
One person only	0.98	(0.81–1.17)
Adult with parents	0.56**	(0.44–0.71)
Adult with one parent	1.23	(0.60–2.11)

* $p<0.05$,   ** $p<0.01$

Table 4.4 Odds ratios of socio–demographic correlates of GP consultations for physical complaint in past year

	Adjusted OR	(95% CI)
Neurotic disorder		
Absent	1.00	....
Present	1.39**	(1.18–1.64)
Physical illness		
Absent	1.00	....
Present	2.91**	(2.32–3.70)
Age		
16–24	1.00	....
25–34	1.00	(0.88–1.14)
35–44	1.13	(0.99–1.30)
45–54	1.20*	(1.04–1.39)
55–64	1.64**	(1.40–1.92)
Sex		
Male	1.00	....
Female	1.35**	(1.23–1.49)
Ethnicity		
White	1.00	....
West Indian or African	1.32	(0.94–1.85)
Asian or Oriental	1.39**	(1.09–1.79)
Other	1.30	(0.81–2.08)
Employment status		
Working full time	1.00	....
Working part time	0.99	(0.87–1.12)
Unemployed	1.07	(0.91–1.26)
Economically inactive	1.26**	(1.12–1.43)
Qualifications		
A level or higher	1.00	....
GCSE/O level	1.12	(1.00–1.25)
Other	1.14	(0.98–1.32)
None	1.21**	(1.08–1.37)
Tenure		
Owner-occupier	1.00	....
Renter	1.14*	(1.02–1.27)

* p<0.05,   ** p<0.01

Table 4.5 Odds ratios of socio–demographic correlates of GP consultations for a mental problem in past year

	Adjusted OR	(95% CI)
Neurotic disorder		
Absent	1.00	....
Present	3.86**	(3.23–4.76)
Physical illness		
Absent	1.00	....
Present	2.40**	(1.92–2.94)
Ethnicity		
White	1.00	....
West Indian or African	1.00	(0.60–1.67)
Asian or Oriental	2.53**	(1.49–4.35)
Other	1.07	(0.51–2.22)
Sex		
Male	1.00	....
Female	1.78**	(1.23–1.49)
Employment status		
Working full time	1.00	....
Working part time	1.41**	(1.15–1.73)
Unemployed	1.62**	(1.27–2.07)
Economically inactive	1.72**	(1.42–2.07)
Drug dependence		
Absent	1.00	....
Present	1.61*	(1.09–2.38)
Age		
16–24	1.00	....
25–34	1.31*	(1.01–1.70)
35–44	1.44**	(1.10–1.90)
45–54	1.58**	(1.20–2.09)
55–64	1.17	(0.87–1.57)

* p<0.05,   ** p<0.01

Table 4.6 Percentage of people with neurotic disorders who had been in-patients in past year, and reason for in-patient stay

	%
In-patient stays for...	
Physical problem	13
Mental problem	1
Mental and physical problem	0
No in-patient stays	86
Base	*1396*

Table 4.7 Number of separate in-patient stays in past 12 months among people with neurotic disorders

Number of stays	%
0	86
1	9
2	3
3 or more	2
Base	*1396*

Table 4.8 Person seen by patient when in hospital for mental health problem

	% of stays involving visit from this professional
Psychiatrist or psychotherapist	31
Other consultant or hospital doctor	25
Occupational therapist	14
Psychiatric nurse	11
Social worker or counsellor	8
Psychologist	6
Other health professional	6
Base (number of stays for which informant stated who they had seen)	*36*

Table 4.9 Number of places visited as out-patient or day patient in past year

Number of places visited	%
0	50
1	34
2	12
3 or more	4
Base	*1396*

55

Table 4.10 Reasons for out-patient or day patient visits by people with neurotic disorders during the past year

		Reason for visit			
		Physical health problem	Mental health problem	Both	*Base*
Women	% visiting	46	5	1	*874*
			50		
Men	% visiting	44	4	1	*521*
			50		
All	% visiting	45	4	1	*1396*
			50		

Table 4.11 Type of place visited by out-patients and day patients for a mental health problem in past year

	% of people with a neurotic disorder visiting establishment
Out-patient department of hospital	55
Private consulting rooms	20
Clinic/Health centre	19
Other	13
Day centre	6
Casualty department of hospital	3
Base (= places visited)	*64*

Table 4.12 Person normally seen at hospital/ clinic by people with neurotic disorders when visiting because of mental health problems

	%
Psychiatrist or psychotherapist	54
Psychologist	19
Other consultant or hospital doctor	13
Psychiatric nurse	13
Social worker or counsellor	12
Other health professional	8
Occupational therapist	6
Base (= places visited)	*64*

Column percentage adds to more than 100% as informants could have seen more than one person

Table 4.13 Source of help which had been turned down by people with neurotic disorders

Source of help	%
Social worker or counselling service	44
Psychiatrist	15
Voluntary worker	8
Home care worker or home help	5
Community psychiatric nurse	4
Occupational therapist	2
Other	3
Not stated	20
Base (= adults who turned down help)	86

Table 4.14 Reason for turning down help or support

	%
Did not want or need help	47
Did not think it could/ would help	27
Could not face it/ handle it	11
Did not like people/ not the right people offering help	6
Inconvenient time or location	3
Other reason	21
Base (= adults who turned down help)	86

Column percentages add to more than 100% because informants could have given more than one reason

Table 4.15 Reason for not seeing a doctor or other professional when others thought they should

	%
Did not think anyone could help	28
A problem one should be able to cope with cope with	28
Did not think it was necessary or no problem	17
Thought problem would get better by itself	14
Too embarrased to discuss it with anyone	13
Afraid of consequences (treatment, tests, hospitalisation, sectioned)	10
Hour inconvenient/did not have time	6
Afraid what family or friends would think	4
Afraid of side effects of any treatment	4
Did not know who to go to or where to go	3
Family or friends objected	1
Other	32
Base	343

Percentages add to more than 100% as people could have given more than one reason

5 Adults with a psychotic disorder

5.1 Introduction

In the previous chapters we have looked at adults with neurotic disorders and how they differed from those without neurotic disorders on various characteristics: socio-demographic attributes, comorbid physical disorders and the use of medication, other forms of treatment, and services. In this chapter, we focus on the relatively small number of adults, forty-four in all, who were identified as having a psychotic disorder.

5.2 Descriptive profile

Adults with a psychotic disorder were equally represented among men and women. About half were aged 16–34 and the largest proportion, 38%, were in the 25–34 age group. Fifty per cent of adults with schizophrenia or bipolar affective disorder were married or cohabiting, 30% were single, and 20% were widowed, divorced or separated. Four in five of those who lived with a partner had at least one child.

About a third of the 44 adults with a psychotic disorder had obtained qualifications at A-level or at a higher level; a similar proportion were in Social Class I, II or III non-manual. In terms of their household characteristics, 49% were living in a terraced house, flat or maisonette; and 78% were living in an urban locality. *(Table 5.1)*.

Because of the relatively small numbers of adults with a psychotic disorder identified from the survey, comparisons with other groups (i.e. those with a neurotic disorder or those with no mental disorder) require caution in their interpretation. Characteristics chosen for comparison in Table 5.2 were selected on the basis that the proportion with a given characteristic among the group with psychosis was about twice that among those with no mental disorder. Thus, compared with adults with no mental disorder, those with a psychotic disorder were about twice as likely to be unemployed or economically inactive, living in rented accommodation, living alone, or divorced or separated. *(Table 5.2)*

5.3 Comorbidity with neurotic disorders and physical illness

All survey respondents were asked the questions from the revised Clinical Interview Schedule (CIS–R). Thus it is possible to look at the neurotic symptomatology of those who were eventually ascribed a psychotic diagnosis.

About two thirds of those with a psychotic disorder obtained a threshold or above score of 12 or more on the CIS–R, and the proportions with a significant score (2 or more) for each of the 14 symptoms of the CIS–R was much closer to that of the neurotic group than those with no mental disorder. *(Table 5.3)*.

Forty per cent of the group with a psychotic illness had a physical illness compared with 50% of those with a neurotic disorder and 30% of those unaffected by any disorder.

5.4 Treatment and use of services

About a half of all the adults identified as having a psychotic disorder were receiving some form of treatment (excluding analgesics). Overall, about a third were on a type of medication which the BNF describes as 'drugs used in psychosis and related conditions'. A third were having therapy or counselling.

Other CNS drugs being used were: anti-cholinergic drugs (20%), antidepressants(10%), and hypnotics (3%). Anti-cholinergic drugs reduce the symptoms of drug induced parkinsonism as the result of taking anti-psychotic drugs. *(Table 5.4)*

The service use profile of adults with a psychotic disorder described in Table 5.5 shows that 82% had received some sort of service in the 12 months prior to interview: two thirds had seen their GP for a 'mental or emotional problem', about a half had attended an out-patient clinic, about a quarter had an in-patient stay and 11% had received a domiciliary visit from a psychiatrist or a community psychiatric nurse.

A whole range and combination of services were used, the majority had seen their GP and had received at least one other service.

Table 5.1 Sociodemographic characteristics of adults with a psychotic disorder

	%		%		%
Age		**Family unit type**		**Tenure**	
16-24	16	Couple, no children	10	Owned outright	7
25-34	38	Couple, with child(ren)	40	Owned with mortgage	34
35-44	15	Lone parent with		Rented from HA or LA	42
45-54	11	child(ren)	12	Rented from other source	17
55-64	21	One person only	31		
		Adult with parents	5		
		Adult with one parent	1	**Type of accommodation**	
Sex				Detached	10
Women	50			Semi-detached	40
Men	50	**Qualifications**		Terraced	22
		A levels or higher	36	Flat or maisonette	27
		GCSE O levels	30		
Ethnicity		Other	10		
White	89	None	24	**Locality**	
West Indian or African	8			Urban	78
Asian or Oriental	1			Semi-rural	17
Other	2	**Employment status**		Rural	5
		Working full time	19		
		Working part time	20		
Marital status		Unemployed	14		
Married	41	Economically inactive	47		
Cohabiting	9				
Single	30	**Social class**			
Widowed	6	I	6		
Divorced	12	II	16		
Separated	2	IIINM	13		
		IIIM	26		
		IV	14		
		V	20		
		Armed forces	1		
		Never worked	4		
Base	*44*	*Base*	*44*	*Base*	*44*

Table 5.2   Characteristics of adults with a psychotic disorder compared with those with a neurotic disorder and those without a mental disorder

	Adults with a psychotic disorder	Adults with a neurotic disorder	Adults with no mental disorder
	Percentage of adults with each characteristic		
Unemployed or economically inactive	61	44	29
In rented accommodation	59	39	25
One-person family	31	18	13
Divorced or separated	14	11	7
Base	*44*	*1557*	*8184*

Table 5.3   Prevalence of CIS-R symptoms by type of mental disorder

	Adults with a psychotic disorder	Adults with a neurotic disorder	Adults with no mental disorder
	Percentage of adults experiencing each symptom		
Fatigue	67	77	17
Sleep problems	59	63	17
Irritability	52	61	14
Worry	56	67	11
Depression	27	43	3
Depressive ideas	39	46	2
Anxiety	28	47	2
Obsessions	34	35	4
Concentration	42	36	3
Somatic symptoms	24	29	3
Compulsions	22	21	4
Phobias	25	22	2
Worry- physical health	19	19	1
Panic	8	15	0
Base	*44*	*1557*	*8184*

Table 5.4 Medication and treatment received by those with a psychotic disorder

	Percentage of adults receiving each type of treatment
Hypnotics and anxiolytics	3
Hypnotics	3
Anxiolytics	-
Drugs used in psychosis and related conditions	34
Anti-psychotic drugs	26
Depot injections	10
Antimanic drugs	10
Antidepressants	10
Tricyclic antidepressants	6
Monoamire oxidose inhibitors	-
Compound antidepressants	-
Serotonin reuptake inhibitors	5
Analgesics	6
Antiepileptics	1
Anticholinergic drugs	20
Any CNS drugs	47
Counselling or therapy	31
Any treatment	57
Base	*44*

Table 5.5 Service use profile

	%
In the past year	
Used no services	18
Seen GP only	18
Seen GP and been an out-patient	17
Out-patient only	14
Seen GP, been in-patient and out-patient	10
Seen GP and been in-patient	8
Seen GP, been in-patient and out-patient, and received domiciliary services	5
Seen GP, been out-patient and received domiciliary services	5
Been an in-patient and out-patient	2
Been an in-patient only	2
Seen GP and received domiciliary visit	1
Base	*44*
Proportion who had seen GP	63
Proportion who had been an out-patient	53
Proportion who had been an in-patient	27
Proportion who had received domiciliary services	11

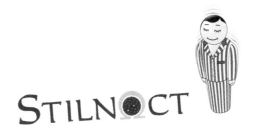

STILNCT

6 Adults with suicidal thoughts

6.1 Introduction

As part of the revised Clinical Interview Schedule, all survey respondents were asked about their experience of depressive symptoms in the seven days prior to interview. Only those with significant symptoms in terms of frequency, severity, or duration were also asked questions relating to depressive ideas including suicidal thoughts. Thus, people with suicidal thoughts that did not have significant depressive symptoms are not included in this chapter. With this proviso, eighty informants, just less than 1% of the overall sample, reported having had thoughts of killing themselves in the seven days prior to the interview.

6.2 Descriptive profile

About two thirds of those who had suicidal thoughts were women, and half were aged 16-34; 28% were aged 16-24. In terms of marital status, just over a third (35%) were married or cohabiting, 36% were single and the remainder (28%) were widowed, divorced or separated. It is therefore not surprising to find that half the sample were either living by themselves or without close relatives, or were lone parents.

A quarter of those who had thought about killing themselves were unemployed and about a half were economically inactive; 11% of this group had never worked.

In terms of household characteristics, 58% were renting; the same proportion was living in a terraced house, flat or maisonette. Overall, 3 in 4 of those with suicidal thoughts were living in an urban locality. *(Table 6.1)*

In comparing the socio-demographic profile of those with suicidal thoughts with the sample

identified as having a neurotic disorder and those unaffected by a mental disorder, marked differences in the proportions with certain characteristics were evident. However it should be noted that standard errors of percentages based on a sample of 80 are far larger than those based on a sample of 8000. Taking this into account, the data in Table 6.2 show that the group of adults with suicidal thoughts were about three times as likely as those with no mental disorder to be widowed, divorced or separated, and also three times more likely to be a lone parent or single person. They were also two and a half times more likely to be unemployed or economically inactive, and to be living in rented accommodation. *(Table 6.2)*

6.3 Neurotic symptoms, neurotic disorders and physical illness

People feeling suicidal often express feelings of worthlessness, hopelessness, self-deprecation, and guilt. All those in the survey who had suicidal thoughts felt life was not worth living, 9 out of 10 had feelings of hopelessness, and at least 8 out of 10 felt "not as good as others", blamed themselves when things went wrong. *(Table 6.3)*

They also scored highly on the 14 symptoms of the CIS-R. Over three quarters scored 2 or more on depression, depressive ideas, worry, irritability or fatigue. *(Table 6.4)*

When the diagnostic algorithms were applied to those with suicidal thoughts, 44% emerged as having 2 or more neurotic disorders, which included 28% with 3 or more disorders. More specifically, 43% were classified as having a depressive episode, 40% with GAD, 28% with mixed anxiety and depressive disorder, 24% with phobia, and 10% with panic. *(Table 6.5)*

Among all groups covered by the survey those with suicidal thoughts had the highest proportion with a physical illness (61%), compared with 50% of those with any neurotic disorder, 40% of adults with a psychotic illness and 30% of those unaffected by a mental disorder.

6.4 Treatment and use of services

About a fifth of those who had thought about killing themselves in the week prior to interview were on antidepressants, the majority, two thirds, were taking tricyclic antidepressants. Twelve per cent of this group were taking hypnotics and anxiolytics, a similar proportion had analgesic medication. About 1 in 6 of the 80 adults identified by the survey as having suicidal thoughts were receiving counselling or therapy. *(Table 6.6)*

The service use profile of those with suicidal thoughts was remarkably similar to that of those adults who had a psychotic disorder both in terms of those who had used each service and the combination of services: about 6 out of 10 had seen their GP in the past year (about half of these in the past week), 5 out of 10 had been an out-patient, about 3 in 10 an in-patient and 1 in 10 had received a domiciliary visit. Overall, 4 in 10 had seen their GP and received at least one other service in the past year. *(Table 6.7)*

Table 6.1 Socio-demographic characteristics of adults with suicidal thoughts

	%		%		%
Age		**Family unit type**		**Tenure**	
16-24	28	Couple, no children	10	Owned outright	4
25-34	22	Couple, with		Owned with mortgage	37
35-44	23	child(ren)	25	Rented from HA or LA	41
45-54	19	Lone parent with		Rented from other source	17
55-64	9	child(ren)	23		
		One person only	28	**Type of accommodation**	
Sex		Adult with parents	12	Detached	15
Women	63	Adult with one parent	2	Semi-detached	27
Men	37			Terraced	25
		Qualifications		Flat or maisonette	33
Ethnicity		A levels or higher	29		
White	88	GCSE O levels	21	**Locality**	
West Indian or African	2	Other	14	Urban	75
Asian or Oriental	8	None	36	Semi-rural	20
Other	2			Rural	5
		Employment status			
Marital status		Working full time	25		
Married	30	Working part time	?		
Cohabiting	5	Unemployed	25		
Single	36	Economically inactive	48		
Widowed	5				
Divorced	15	**Social class**			
Separated	8	I	3		
		II	16		
		IIINM	18		
		IIIM	26		
		IV	17		
		V	4		
		Armed forces	2		
		Never worked	11		
Base	*80*	*Base*	*80*	*Base*	*80*

Table 6.2   Characteristics of adults with suicidal thoughts compared with those with a neurotic disorder and without a mental disorder

	Adults with suicidal thoughts		Adults with a neurotic disorder		Adults with no neurotic disorder	
Percentage of adults with each characteristic						
Widowed	5		4		2	
Divorced	15	28	8	15	5	9
Separated	8		3		2	
Lone parent and child(ren)	23		10		5	
		51		28		18
One person only	28		18		13	
Unemployed	25		14		9	
Economically inactive	48	73	30	44	21	29
(Never worked)	11		2		2	
Rented from HA or LA	41		28		16	
		58		39		25
Rented from other source	17		11		9	
Base	*80*		*1557*		*8484*	

Table 6.3   Depressive ideas of those with suicidal thoughts

	Percentage who had each depressive idea in the 7 days prior to interview
Feeling sad, miserable or depressed made them...	
Feel very restless	63
Do things slowly	68
Be less talkative	82
Blamed themselves when things went wrong	83
Felt not as good as others	82
Had feelings of hopelessness	90
Felt life was not worth living	100
Base	*80*

Table 6.4 Prevalence of CIS-R symptoms of those with suicidal thoughts

	Adults with suicidal thoughts	Adults with a neurotic disorder	Adults with no mental disorder
	Percentage of adults experiencing each symptom		
Fatigue	77	77	17
Sleep problems	71	63	17
Irritability	80	61	14
Worry	85	67	11
Depression	77	43	3
Depressive ideas	100	46	2
Anxiety	66	47	2
Obsessions	59	35	4
Concentration & forgetfulness	56	36	3
Somatic symptoms	43	29	3
Compulsions	38	20	4
Phobias	38	22	2
Worry- physical health	36	19	1
Panic	32	15	0
Base	*80*	*1557*	*8184*

Table 6.5 Proportion of adults with suicidal thoughts having each neurotic disorder

	Percentage with each neurotic disorder
Mixed anxiety and depressive disorder	28
Generalised Anxiety Disorder	40
Depressive episode	
mild	2
moderate	16
severe	25
All	43
Phobia	
agoraphobia	12
social	5
specific	7
All	24
Obsessive-Compulsive Disorder	28
Panic	10
Base	*80*

Summary: number of neurotic disorders	%
None*	4
1	52
2	16
3	23
4	5

* Had a psychotic disorder

65

Table 6.6 Medication and treatment received by those with suicidal thoughts

	Percentage of adults receiving each type of treatment
Hypnotics and anxiolytics	12
Hypnotics	5
Anxiolytics	8
Drugs used in psychosis and related conditions	3
Antidepressants	21
Tricyclic antidepressants	14
Monoamine oxidase inhibitor	-
Compound antidepressants	-
Serotonin reuptake inhibitors	8
Drugs used in nausea and vertigo	1
Analgesics	12
Non-opioid analgesics	8
Opioid analgesics	4
Antiepileptics	4
Anticholinergic drugs	2
Drugs used in substance abuse	1
Any CNS drugs	38
Counselling or therapy	17
Any treatment	42
Base	*80*

Table 6.7 Service use profile

	%
In the past year	
Used no services	20
Seen GP only	17
Seen GP and been an out-patient	16
Out-patient only	16
Seen GP, been in-patient and out-patient	10
Seen GP and been an in-patient	5
Seen GP, been in-patient, out-patient and received domiciliary visits	4
Been an in-patient and out-patient	4
Been an in-patient only	2
Seen GP and received domiciliary visits	2
Seen GP, been an out-patient and received domiciliary visits	2
Seen GP, been an in-patient and received domiciliary visits	1
Base	*80*
Proportion who had seen GP	58
Proportion who had been an out-patient	50
Proportion who had been an in-patient	27
Proportion who had received domiciliary services	9

Appendices and Glossary

Appendix A: Measuring psychiatric morbidity

A1 Identifying neurotic psychopathology

To obtain the prevalence of both symptoms and diagnoses of neurotic psychopathology, the revised version of the Clinical Interview Schedule (CIS–R) was chosen.[1] The CIS–R is made up of 14 sections, each section covering a particular area of neurotic symptoms.

Each section within the interview schedule starts with a variable number of mandatory questions which can be regarded as sift or filter questions. They establish the existence of a particular neurotic symptom in the past month. A positive response to these questions leads the interviewer on to further enquiry giving a more detailed assessment of the symptom in the past week. The symptom is assessed in terms of frequency, duration, severity and time since onset. The informant's responses to these questions determine the score on each section. More frequent and more severe symptoms result in higher scores.

The minimum score on each section is 0, where the symptom was either not present in the past week or was present only in mild degree. The maximum score on each section is 4 (except for the section on Depressive ideas which has a maximum score of 5).

- Summed scores from all 14 sections range between 0 and 57.
- The overall threshold score for significant psychiatric morbidity is 12.
- Symptoms are regarded as significant if they have a score of 2 or more.

The elements contributing to scores on each symptom are shown below:

Fatigue
Scores relate to fatigue or feeling tired or lacking in energy in the past week.
Score one for each of:
- Symptom present on four days or more
- Symptom present for more than three hours in total on any day
- Subject had to push him/herself to get things done on at least one occasion
- Symptom present when subject doing things he/she enjoys or used to enjoy at least once

Sleep problems
Scores relate to problems with getting to sleep, or otherwise, with sleeping more than is usual for the subject in the past week.
Score one for each of:
- Had problems with sleep for four nights or more
- Spent at least 4 hours trying to get to sleep on the night with least sleep
- Spent at least 1 hour trying to get to sleep on the night with least sleep
- Spent three hours or more trying to get to sleep on four nights or more
- Slept for at least 4 hours longer than usual for subject on any night
- Slept for at least 1 hour longer than usual for subject on any night
- Slept for more than three hours longer than usual for subject on four nights or more

Irritability
Scores relate to feelings of irritability, being short-tempered or angry in the past week.
Score one for each of:
- Symptom present for four days or more
- Symptom present for more than one hour on any day
- Wanted to shout at someone (even if subject had not actually shouted)
- Had arguments, rows or quarrels or lost temper with someone and felt it was unjustified on at least one occasion

Worry
Scores relate to subject's experience of worry in the past week, other than worry about physical health.
Score one for each of:
- Symptom present on four or more days
- Has been worrying too much in view of circumstances
- Symptom has been very unpleasant
- Symptom lasted over three hours in total on any day

Depression
Applies to subjects who felt sad, miserable or depressed or unable to enjoy or take an interest in things as much as usual, in the past week. Scores relate to the subject's experience in the past week.
Score one for each of:
- Unable to enjoy or take an interest in things as much as usual

- Symptom present on four days or more
- Symptom lasted for more than three hours in total on any day
- When sad, miserable or depressed subject did not become happier when something nice happened, or when in company

Depressive ideas
Applies to subjects who had a score of 1 for depression. Scores relate to experience in the past week.
Score one for each of:
- Felt guilty or blamed him/herself at least once when things went wrong when it had not been his/her fault
- Felt not as good as other people
- Felt hopeless
- Felt that life isn't worth living
- Thought of killing him/herself

Anxiety
Scores relate to feeling generally anxious, nervous or tense in the past week. These feelings were not the result of a phobia.
Score one for each of:
- Symptom present on four or more days
- Symptom had been very unpleasant
- When anxious, nervous or tense, had one or more of following symptoms:
    heart racing or pounding
    hands sweating or shaking
    feeling dizzy
    difficulty getting breath
    butterflies in stomach
    dry mouth
    nausea or feeling as though he/she wanted to vomit
- Symptom present for more than three hours in total on any one day

Obsessions
Scores relate to the subject's experience of having repetitive unpleasant thoughts or ideas in the past week.
Score one for each of:
- Symptom present on four or more days
- Tried to stop thinking any of these thoughts
- Became upset or annoyed when had these thoughts
- Longest episode of the symptom was $\frac{1}{4}$ hour or longer

Concentration and forgetfulness
Scores relate to the subject's experience of concentration problems and forgetfulness in the past week.
Score one for each of:
- Symptoms present for four days or more
- Could not always concentrate on a TV programme, read a newspaper article or talk to someone

without mind wandering
- Problems with concentration stopped subject from getting on with things he/she used to do or would have liked to do
- Forgot something important

Somatic symptoms
Scores relate to the subject's experience in the past week of any ache, pain or discomfort which was brought on or made worse by feeling low, anxious or stressed.
Score one for each of:
- Symptom present for four days or more
- Symptom lasted more than three hours on any day
- Symptom had been very unpleasant
- Symptom bothered subject when doing something interesting

Compulsions
Scores relate to the subject's experience of doing things over again when subject had already done them in the past week.
Score one for each of:
- Symptom present on four days or more
- Subject tried to stop repeating behaviour
- Symptom made subject upset or annoyed with him/herself
- Repeated behaviour three or more times when it had already been done

Phobias
Scores relate to subject's experience of phobias or avoidance in the past week
Score one for each of:
- Felt nervous/anxious about a situation or thing four or more times
- On occasions when felt anxious, nervous or tense, had one or more of following symptoms:
    heart racing or pounding
    hands sweating or shaking
    feeling dizzy
    difficulty getting breath
    butterflies in stomach
    dry mouth
    nausea or feeling as though he/she wanted to vomit
- Avoided situation or thing at least once because it would have made subject anxious, nervous or tense
- Avoided situation or thing four times or more because it would have made subject anxious, nervous or tense

Worry about physical health
Scores relate to experience of the symptom in the past week.
Score one for each of:
- Symptom present on four days or more
- Subject felt he/she had been worrying too much in view of actual health

- Symptom had been very unpleasant
- Subject could not be distracted by doing something else

Panic

Applies to subjects who felt anxious, nervous or tense in the past week and the scores relate to the resultant feelings of panic, or of collapsing and losing control in the past week.

Score one for each of:
- Symptom experienced once
- Symptom experienced more than once
- Symptom had been very unpleasant or unbearable
- An episode lasted longer than 10 minutes

Any combination of the elements produce the section score.

As well as having certain significant symptoms, other criteria had to be met for a neurotic diagnosis to be obtained. The algorithms for identifying each disorder are shown below.

Algorithms for production of ICD-10 diagnoses of neurosis from the CIS-R ('scores' refer to CIS-R scores)

F32.00 Mild depressive episode without somatic symptoms

1. Symptom duration ≥ 2 weeks

2. *Two or more from:*

   - depressed mood
   - loss of interest
   - fatigue

3. *Two or three from:*

   - reduced concentration
   - reduced self-esteem
   - ideas of guilt
   - pessimism about future
   - suicidal ideas or acts
   - disturbed sleep
   - diminished appetite

4. Social impairment

5. *Fewer than four from:*

   - lack of normal pleasure /interest
   - loss of normal emotional reactivity
   - a.m. waking ≥ 2 hours early
   - loss of libido
   - diurnal variation in mood
   - diminished appetite
   - loss of ≥ 5% body weight
   - psychomotor agitation
   - psychomotor retardation

F32.01 Mild depressive episode with somatic symptoms

1. Symptom duration ≥ 2 weeks

2. *Two or more from:*

   - depressed mood
   - loss of interest
   - fatigue

3. *Two or three from:*

   - reduced concentration
   - reduced self-esteem
   - ideas of guilt
   - pessimism about future
   - suicidal ideas or acts
   - disturbed sleep
   - diminished appetite

4. Social impairment

5. *Four or more from:*

   - lack of normal pleasure /interest
   - loss of normal emotional reactivity
   - a.m. waking ≥ 2 hours early
   - loss of libido
   - diurnal variation in mood
   - diminished appetite
   - loss of ≥5% body weight
   - psychomotor agitation
   - psychomotor retardation

F32.10 Moderate depressive episode without somatic symptoms

1. Symptom duration ≥2 weeks

2. *Two or more* from:

   - depressed mood
   - loss of interest
   - fatigue

3. *Four or more* from:

   - reduced concentration
   - reduced self-esteem
   - ideas of guilt
   - pessimism about future
   - suicidal ideas or acts

- disturbed sleep
- diminished appetite

4. Social impairment

5. *Fewer than four* from:

- lack of normal pleasure/interest
- loss of normal emotional reactivity
- a.m. waking ≥ 2 hours early
- loss of libido
- diurnal variation in mood
- diminished appetite
- loss of ≥ 5% body weight
- psychomotor agitation
- psychomotor retardation

F32.11 Moderate depressive episode with somatic symptoms

1. Symptom duration ≥2 weeks

2. *Two or more* from:

- depressed mood
- loss of interest
- fatigue

3. *Four or more* from:

- reduced concentration
- reduced self-esteem
- ideas of guilt
- pessimism about future
- suicidal ideas or acts
- disturbed sleep
- diminished appetite

4. Social impairment

5. *Four or more* from:

- lack of normal pleasure /interest
- loss of normal emotional reactivity
- a.m. waking ≥2 hours early
- loss of libido
- diurnal variation in mood
- diminished appetite
- loss of ≥ 5% body weight
- psychomotor agitation
- psychomotor retardation

F32.2 Severe depressive episode

1. *All three* from:

- depressed mood
- loss of interest
- fatigue

2. *Four or more* from:

- reduced concentration
- reduced self-esteem
- ideas of guilt
- pessimism about future
- suicidal ideas or acts
- disturbed sleep
- diminished appetite

3. Social impairment

4. *Four or more* from:

- lack of normal pleasure /interest
- loss of normal emotional reactivity
- a.m. waking ≥ 2 hours early
- loss of libido
- diurnal variation in mood
- diminished appetite
- loss of ≥ 5% body weight
- psychomotor agitation
- psychomotor retardation

F40.00 Agoraphobia without panic disorder
1. Fear of open spaces and related aspects: crowds, distance from home, travelling alone
2. Social impairment
3. Avoidant behaviour must be prominent feature
4. Overall phobia score ≥ 2
5. No panic attacks

F40.01 Agoraphobia with panic disorder
1. Fear of open spaces and related aspects: crowds, distance from home, travelling alone
2. Social impairment
3. Avoidant behaviour must be prominent feature
4. Overall phobia score ≥ 2
5. Panic disorder (overall panic score ≥ 2)

F40.1 Social phobias
1. Fear of scrutiny by other people: eating or speaking in public etc.
2. Social impairment
3. Avoidant behaviour must be prominent feature
4. Overall phobia score ≥ 2

F40.2 Specific (isolated) phobias
1. Fear of specific situations or things, e.g. animals, insects, heights, blood, flying, etc.
2. Social impairment
3. Avoidant behaviour must be prominent feature
4. Overall phobia score ≥ 2

F41.0 Panic disorder
1. Criteria for phobic disorders not met
2. Recent panic attacks
3. Anxiety-free between attacks
4. Overall panic score ≥ 2

F41.1 Generalised Anxiety Disorder
1. Duration $\geq$ 6 months
2. Free-floating anxiety
3. Autonomic overactivity
4. Overall anxiety score $\geq$ 2

F41.2 Mixed anxiety and depressive disorder
1. (Sum of scores for each CIS-R section) $\geq$ 12
2. Criteria for other categories not met

F42 Obsessive-Compulsive Disorder
1. Duration $\geq$ 2 weeks
2. At least one act/thought resisted
3. Social impairment
4. Overall scores:
   obsession score=4, or
   compulsion score=4, or
   obsession+compulsion scores $\geq$ 6

Those with CIS–R scores of 12 or more, who did not fit the criteria for any of the nine neurotic disorders listed above, were categorised as having mixed anxiety and depressive disorder.

A2 Identifying psychotic psycho-pathology

A sift interview was conducted using an instrument specifically designed for this survey, the psychosis screening questionnaire.[2] Once those with a potential psychotic disorder had been identified, Schizophrenia and other functional psychoses were derived from SCAN[3] interviews by clinicians. A diagnosis of 'psychosis unspecified' was also made on the basis of data collected by OPCS interviewers when clinical assessments could not be made.

A3 Obtaining the classification system of different disorders

The survey identified three psychotic and nine specific neurotic disorders from SCAN and CIS–R results, based on ICD–10 diagnostic criteria.[4]

The psychotic disorders were combined in one group and the neurotic disorders were grouped into 6 diagnostic classes for most analysis. The derivation of the various disorders and the way in which the information was analysed is shown below.

Although it was possible for individuals to have more than one disorder, in Report 1 each individual was classified according to their most severe, or primary disorder. The hierarchy used to determine the primary disorder is shown below.

Primary disorder hierarchy used for prevalence estimates in Report 1 (disorders listed in descending order of severity)

A   Any psychotic disorder

B   Neurotic disorders as follows:

1   **severe depressive episode**
2   **moderate depressive episode**
3   **panic disorder**
4   **Obsessive–Compulsive Disorder (OCD)**
5   **mild depressive episode**
6   **social phobia**
7   **agoraphobia**
8   **Generalised Anxiety Disorder (GAD)**
9   **specific isolated phobia**
10 **mixed anxiety and depressive disorder**

Once the most severe disorder had been identified, some of the categories were collapsed such that severe, moderate and mild depressive episode were grouped under 'depressive episode' and social phobia, agoraphobia and specific isolated phobia were described collectively as 'phobias'.

Notes and references

1.   Lewis, G. and Pelosi, A. J., *Manual of the Revised Clinical Interview Schedule, (CIS–R)*, June 1990, Institute of Psychiatry.

     Lewis, G., Pelosi, A.J., Araya, R.C. and Dunn, G., (1992) Measuring psychiatric disorder in the community: a standardized assessment for use by lay interviewers, *Psychological Medicine*, 22, 465–486

2.   Bebbington, P.E., and Nayani, T (1995). The psychosis screening questionnaire. *International Journal of Methods in Psychiatric Research*. Volume 5:11–19

3.   *Schedules for Clinical Assessment in Neuropsychiatry*, 1992, WHO, Division of Mental Health, Geneva

4.   *WHO, The ICD–10 Classification of Mental and Behavioural Disorders: Diagnostic Criteria for Research*: 1993, WHO, Geneva.

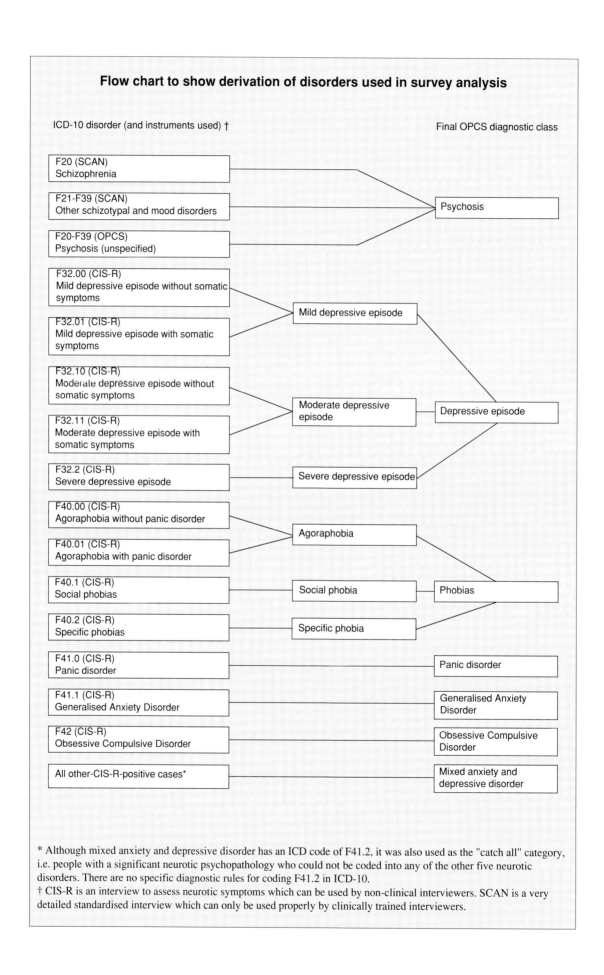

Flow chart to show derivation of disorders used in survey analysis

ICD-10 disorder (and instruments used) †

Final OPCS diagnostic class

F20 (SCAN)
Schizophrenia

F21-F39 (SCAN)
Other schizotypal and mood disorders

F20-F39 (OPCS)
Psychosis (unspecified)

Psychosis

F32.00 (CIS-R)
Mild depressive episode without somatic symptoms

F32.01 (CIS-R)
Mild depressive episode with somatic symptoms

Mild depressive episode

F32.10 (CIS-R)
Moderate depressive episode without somatic symptoms

F32.11 (CIS-R)
Moderate depressive episode with somatic symptoms

Moderate depressive episode

Depressive episode

F32.2 (CIS-R)
Severe depressive episode

Severe depressive episode

F40.00 (CIS-R)
Agoraphobia without panic disorder

F40.01 (CIS-R)
Agoraphobia with panic disorder

Agoraphobia

F40.1 (CIS-R)
Social phobias

Social phobia

Phobias

F40.2 (CIS-R)
Specific phobias

Specific phobia

F41.0 (CIS-R)
Panic disorder

Panic disorder

F41.1 (CIS-R)
Generalised Anxiety Disorder

Generalised Anxiety Disorder

F42 (CIS-R)
Obsessive Compulsive Disorder

Obsessive Compulsive Disorder

All other-CIS-R-positive cases*

Mixed anxiety and depressive disorder

* Although mixed anxiety and depressive disorder has an ICD code of F41.2, it was also used as the "catch all" category, i.e. people with a significant neurotic psychopathology who could not be coded into any of the other five neurotic disorders. There are no specific diagnostic rules for coding F41.2 in ICD-10.
† CIS-R is an interview to assess neurotic symptoms which can be used by non-clinical interviewers. SCAN is a very detailed standardised interview which can only be used properly by clinically trained interviewers.

Appendix B Multiple logistic regression (MLR) and Odds Ratios (OR)

B1 Interpretation of odds ratios

Chapters 2 to 4 of this report use logistic regression analysis to provide a measure of the effect of having a neurotic disorder on for example having seen a GP in the past 2 weeks. Unlike many of the crosstabulations presented elsewhere in the report, MLR estimates the effect of a neurotic disorder while controlling for the confounding effect of other variables in the analysis. A forward stepwise method of logistic regression was used. The dependent variable was dichotomous, indicating the presence or absence of a particular behaviour or state. All variables were categorical

Logistic regression produces an estimate of the probability of an event occurring when an individual is in a particular category of a sociodemographic variable compared to a reference category of that variable. The odds of the event occurring are defined as the ratio of the probability of the event occurring compared with its absence. If the probability of an event is p, the odds are $p/(1-p)$. The factor by which the odds of an event differ for people in a particular category compared with those in the reference category is shown by the adjusted odds ratio (OR). The OR controls for the possible confounding effects of other variables in the statistical model, for example, sex, age and employment status. To determine whether this increased odds of the event occurring are due to chance rather than to the effect of the variable, one must consult the confidence interval associated with the odds ratio.

B2 Confidence intervals around an odds ratio

In Table 4.3, for example, an odds ratio of 1.86 is shown with a confidence interval from 1.54 to 2.22, indicating that the 'true' (i.e. population) OR is 95% likely to lie between these two values. If the confidence interval does not include 1.00 then the OR is likely to be significantly different from the reference category.

B3 Significance

It is stated in the text of the report that some odds ratios are 'significant'. This indicates that it is unlikely that an odds ratio of this magnitude would be found due to chance alone. Specifically, the likelihood that the OR shows an effect simply by chance is less than 5%. This is conventionally assumed to be infrequent enough to discount chance as an explanation for the finding.

Glossary of survey definitions and terms

Adults
In this survey adults were defined as persons aged 16 or over and less than aged 65.

Alcohol dependence
This was derived from responses to a self-completion questionnaire asked of all survey respondents. An individual was classified as alcohol dependent if they had three or more positive responses to the following twelve statements.

Loss of control

1. Once I started drinking it was difficult for me to stop before I became completely drunk

2. I sometimes kept on drinking after I had promised myself not to.

3. I deliberately tried to cut down or stop drinking, but I was unable to do so.

4. Sometimes I have needed a drink so badly that I could not think of anything else.

Symptomatic behaviour

5. I have skipped a number of regular meals while drinking

6. I have often had an alcoholic drink the first thing when I got up in the morning.

7. I have had a strong drink in the morning to get over the previous night's drinking

8. I have woken up the next day not being able to remember some of the things I had done while drinking.

9. My hand shook a lot in the morning after drinking.

10. I need more alcohol than I used to get the same effect as before.

11. Sometimes I have woken up during the night or early morning sweating all over because of drinking.

Binge Drinking

12. I have stayed drunk for several days at a time.

Antipsychotic drugs
These are also known as 'neuroleptics'. In the short term they are used to quieten disturbed patients whatever the underlying psychopathology.
See Depot Injections

Depot injections
When antipsychotic medication is given by injections on a monthly basis, these are sometimes termed depot injections.

Drug dependence
This was derived from responses to a self-completion questionnaire asked of all survey respondents. An individual was classified as drug dependent if they had a positive response to any of the following five questions in relation to the 10 drugs listed in the box below. A prerequisite was that the drug(s) must have been taken either without a prescription, more than was prescribed for the subject, or to get high.

---

1. Sleeping Pills, Barbiturates, Sedatives, Downers, Seconal
2. Tranquillisers, Valium, Librium
3. Cannabis, Marijuana, Hash, Dope, Grass, Ganja, Kif
4. Amphetamines, Speed, Uppers, Stimulants, Qat
5. Cocaine, Coke, Crack
6. Heroin, Smack
7. Opiates other than herion: Demerol, Morphine, Methadone, Darvon, Opium, DF118
8. Psychedelics, Hallucinogens: LSD, Mescaline, Acid, Peyote, Psylocybin (Magic) mushrooms
9. Ecstasy
0. Solvents, inhalants, glue, amyl nitrate

---

1. Have you ever used any one of these drugs every day for two weeks or more in the past twelve months?

2. In the past twelve months have you used any one of these drugs to the extent that you felt like you needed it or were dependent on it?

3. In the past twelve months, have you tried to cut down on any drugs but found you could not do it?

4. In the past twelve months did you find that you needed larger amounts of these drugs to get an effect, or that you could no longer get high on the amount you used to use?

5. In the past twelve months have you had withdrawal symptoms such as feeling sick because you stopped or cut down on any of these drugs?

Educational level

Educational level was based on the highest educational qualification obtained and was grouped as follows:

Degree (or degree level qualification)

Teaching, HND, Nursing
  Teaching qualification
  HNC/HND, BEC/TEC Higher, BTEC Higher
  City and Guilds Full Technological
   Certificate
  Nursing qualifications:
  (SRN,SCM,RGN,RM,RHV,
  Midwife)

A level
  GCE A-levels/SCE higher
  ONC/OND/BEC/TEC/not higher
  City and Guilds Advanced/Final level
O level
  GCE O-level (grades A-C if after 1975)
  GCSE (grades A-C)
  CSE (grade 1)
  SCE Ordinary (bands A-C)
  Standard grade (levels 1-3)
  SLC Lower SUPE Lower or Ordinary
  School certificate or Matric
  City and Guilds Craft/Ordinary level

GCSE/CSE
  GCE O-level (grades D-E if after 1975)
  GCSE (grades D-G)
  CSE (grades 2-5)
  SCE Ordinary (bands D-E)
  Standard grade (levels 4-5)

  Clerical or commercial qualifications
  Apprenticeship
  Other qualifications

No qualifications
  CSE ungraded
  No qualifications

Employment status

Four types of employment status were identified: working full time, working part time, unemployed and economically inactive.

Working adults

The two categories of working adults include persons who did any work for pay or profit in the week ending the last Sunday prior to interview, even if it was for as little as one hour, including Saturday jobs and casual work (e.g. babysitting, running a mail order club).

Self-employed persons were considered to be working if they worked in their own business, professional practice, or farm for the purpose of making a profit, or even if the enterprise was failing to make a profit or just being set up.

The unpaid 'family worker' (e.g., a wife doing her husband's accounts or helping with the farm or business) was included as working if the work contributed directly to a business, farm or family practice owned or operated by a related member of the same household. (Although the individual concerned may have received no pay or profit, her contribution to the business profit counted as paid work.) This only applied when the business was owned or operated by a member of the same household.

Anyone on a Government scheme which was employer based was also 'working last week'.

Informants' definitions dictated whether they felt they were working full time or part time.

Unemployed adults

This category included those who were waiting to take up a job that had already been obtained, those who were looking for work, and people who intended to look for work but were prevented by temporary ill-health, sickness or injury. 'Temporary' was defined by the informant.

Economically inactive

This category comprised five main categories of people:

'Going to school or college' only applied to people

who were under 50 years of age. The category included people following full-time educational courses at school or at further education establishments (colleges, university, etc). It included all school children (16 years and over).

During vacations, students were treated as 'going to school or college' even where their return to college was dependent on passing a set of exams. If however, they were having a break from full-time education, i.e. they were taking a year out, they were not counted as being in full-time education.

'Permanently unable to work because of long-term sickness or disability' only applied to those under state retirement age, ie to men aged 16 to 64 and to women aged 16 to 59. 'Permanently' and 'long-term' were defined by the informant.

'Retired' only applied to those who retired from their full-time occupation at age 50 or over and were not seeking further employment of any kind.

'Looking after the home or family' covered anyone who was mainly involved in domestic duties, provided this person had not already been coded in an earlier category.

'Doing something else' included anyone for whom the earlier categories were inappropriate.

Ethnicity
Household members were classified into nine groups by the person answering Schedule A.

White	White
Black - Caribbean Black - African Black - Other	West Indian/African
Indian Pakistani Bangladeshi Chinese	Asian/Oriental
None of these	Other

For analysis purpose these nine groups were subsumed under 4 headings: White, West Indian/African, Asian/Oriental and Other.

Family unit
In order to classify the relationships of the subject to other members of the households, the household members were divided into family units.

Subjects were assigned to a family unit depending on whether they were or ever had been married, and whether they (or their partners) had any children living with them.

A 'child' was defined for family unit purposes as an adult who lives with one or two parents, provided he or she has never been married and has no child of his or her own in the household.

For example, a household containing three women, a grandmother, mother and child would contain two family units with the mother and child being in one unit, and the grandmother being in another. Hence family units can consist of:

- A married or cohabiting couple or a lone parent with their children

- Other married or cohabiting couples

- An adult who has previously been married. If the adult is now living with parents, the parents are treated as being in a separate family unit

- An adult who does not live with either a spouse, partner, child or parent. This can include adults who live with siblings or with other unrelated people, e.g. flatmates.

Family unit type
Each informant's family unit was classified into one of six family unit types:

'Couple no children' included a married or cohabiting couple without children.

'Couple with child' comprised a married or cohabiting couple with at least one child from their liaison or any previous relationship.

'Lone parent' describes both men and women (who may be single, widowed, divorced or separated) living with at least one child. The subject in this case could be a divorced man looking after his 12 year-old son or a 55 year-old widow looking after a 35 year-old, daughter who had never married and had no children of her own.

'One person' describes the family unit type and does not necessarily mean living alone. It includes people living alone but includes one person living with a sister, or the grandmother who is living with her daughter and her family. It also includes adults living with unrelated people in shared houses, e.g. flatmates.

'Adult living with parents' describes a family unit which has the same members as 'couple with child' but in this case it is the adult son or daughter who is the subject. It includes a 20 year old unmarried student living at home with married or cohabiting parents, and a 62 year old single woman caring for her elderly parents.

'Adult living with lone parent' covers the same situations as above except that there is one and not two parents in the household.

Household

The standard definition used in most surveys carried out by OPCS Social Survey Division, and comparable with the 1991 Census definition of a household, was used in this survey. A household is defined as a single person or group of people who have the accommodation as their only or main residence and who either share one meal a day or share the living accommodation. (See E McCrossan *A Handbook for interviewers*. HMSO: London 1985.)

Locality

Interviewers coded their opinion of whether the sampled address was in an urban, semi-rural or rural area.

Marital status

Informants were categorised according to their own perception of marital status. Married and cohabiting took priority over other categories. Cohabiting included anyone living together with their partner as a couple.

Perceived social support

The level of social support which informants reported was based on responses to the following 7 statements. Respondents could say that each statement was not true, partly true or certainly true.

There are people I know – amongst my family or friends – who...

1. do things to make me happy
2. make me feel loved
3. can be relied on no matter what happens
4. would see that I am taken care of if I needed to be
5. accept me just as I am
6. make me feel an important part of their lives
7. give me support and encouragement

Each response of not true scored 1, party true scored 2 and certainly true scored 3; individuals therefore had a total score of between 7 and 21.

Social support was classified as:

> severe lack (scores 7 to 17)
> moderate lack (scores 18 to 20)
> no lack (score 21)

Physical complaints

Informants were asked 'Do you have any long-standing illness, disability or infirmity? By long-standing I mean anything that has troubled you over a period of time or that is likely to affect you over a period of time?'

Those that answered yes to this question were then asked 'What is the matter with you?'; interviewers were asked to try and obtain a medical diagnosis, or to establish the main symptoms. From these responses, illnesses were coded to the site or system of the body that was affected, using a classification system that roughly corresponded to the chapter headings of the International Classification of Diseases (ICD–10). Some of the illnesses identified were mental illnesses and these were excluded from the classification of physical illness. Physical illness did, however, include physical disabilities and sensory complaints such as eyesight and hearing problems.

Psychiatric morbidity

The expression psychiatric morbidity refers to the degree or extent of the prevalence of mental health problems within a defined area.

Region

When the survey was carried out there were 14 Regional Health authorities in England. These were the basis for stratified sampling and have been retained for purposes of analysis. Scotland and Wales were treated as two distinct areas.

Social class

Based on the Registrar General's 1991 *Standard Occupational Classification,* Volume 3 OPCS, HMSO: London social class was ascribed on the basis of the following priorities:

Firstly, social class was based on the informant's own occupation, unless the informant was a married or cohabiting woman. In such cases, the spouse or partner's occupation was used. The exception is where the spouse or partner had never worked, in which case the woman's own occupation was used.

Secondly, social class was based on the informant' (or spouse's) current occupation or, if the informant (or spouse) was unemployed or economically inactive at the time of interview but had previously worked, social class was based on the most recent previous occupation.

The classification used in the tables is as follows:

Descriptive definition	Social class
Professional	I
Intermediate occupations	II
Skilled occupations — non-manual	III NM
Skilled occupations — manual	III M
Partly-skilled	IV
Unskilled occupations	V
Armed Forces	

Social class was not determined where the subject (and spouse) had never worked, or if the subject was a full-time student or where occupation was inadequately described.

Stressful life events
Responses of 'yes' to any of the following 11 questions identified a recent stressful life event.

In the past 6 months...

1. have you yourself suffered from a serious illness, injury or an assault?

2. has a serious illness, injury or an assault happened to a close relative?

3. has a parent, spouse (or partner), child, brother or sister of yours died?

4. has a close family friend or another relative died, such as an aunt, cousin or grandparent?

5. have you had a separation due to marital difficulties or broken off a steady relationship?

6. have you had a serious problem with a close friend, neighbour or relative?

7. were you made redundant or sacked from your job?

8. were you seeking work without success for more than one month?

9. did you have a major financial crisis, such as losing the equivalent of 3 months income?

10. did you have problems with the police involving a court appearance?

11. was something you valued lost or stolen?

Informants were classified according to the number of stressful life events they had experienced in the last 6 months.

Tenure
Four tenure categories were created:

'Owned outright' means bought without mortgage or loan or with a mortgage or loan which has been paid off.

'Owned with mortgage' includes co-ownership and shared ownership schemes.

'Rent from LA/HA' means rented from local authorities, New Town corporations or commissions or Scottish Homes, and housing associations which include co-operatives and property owned by charitable trusts.

'Rent from other source' includes rent from organisations (property company, employer or other organisation) and from individuals (relative, friend, employer or other individual).

Printed in the United Kingdom for HMSO.
Dd.0301845, 12/95, C20, 3400, 5673, 340345.

81